# Ophthalmology of Exotic Pets

# Ophthalmology of Exotic Pets

## David L. Williams

MA VetMB PhD CertVOphthal CertWEL FHEA FSB FRCVS

*Associate Lecturer in Veterinary Ophthalmology*
*Department of Clinical Veterinary Medicine*
*University of Cambridge, UK*

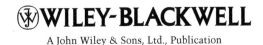

A John Wiley & Sons, Ltd., Publication

*Library of Congress Cataloging-in-Publication Data*

Williams, David L., MA.
  Ophthalmology of exotic pets / David L. Williams.
      p. ; cm.
  Includes bibliographical references and index.
  ISBN 978-1-4443-3041-0 (pbk. : alk. paper)
  I. Title.
  [DNLM: 1. Eye Diseases–veterinary–Handbooks. 2. Pets–Handbooks. SF 891]
  LC classification not assigned
  636.089'77–dc23
                                            2011034163

A catalogue record for this book is available from the British Library.

Wiley also publishes its books in a variety of electronic formats. Some content that appears in print may not be available in electronic books.

Set in 10/12.5 pt Times by Toppan Best-set Premedia Limited

1   2012

Line illustrations by Samantha Elmhurst

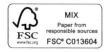

# Contents

# Foreword

The light of the body is the eye: therefore when thine eye is single, thy whole body also is full of light: but when thine eye is evill, thy body also is full of darkenesse.

*Gospel of St Luke 11: 34. King James Version (1611)*

The importance of the eye, in terms of health, is emphasised in the quotation above. St Luke is believed to have been a physician. The eye in its different forms has long attracted interest and attention.

In geological time light-sensitive structures appeared long before the vertebrate eye. Photoreceptors in single-celled organisms permitted the latter to be aware of light and, if necessary, to respond to it by moving or changing behaviour (photoperiodism) but the cells were not sufficiently complex to facilitate detailed navigation nor, indeed, to interpret light in any detail. Simple photoreception has, however, enabled many extinct and extant single-celled organisms to take maximum advantage of sunlight for photosynthesis and move towards it. Insofar as complex eyes are concerned, fossils representing the early appearance of such date back 500–550 million years ago, to the period of rapid evolutionary change that is commonly called the 'Cambrian Explosion'. This resulted in the appearance of a wide range of ocular structures, which differed in acuity, the range of wavelengths that they could detect and whether they could differentiate colours.

The origin and evolution of the eye has attracted much scientific investigation and, interestingly, both academic and public debate. The detail and apparent sophistication of the mammalian eye even prompted Charles Darwin at one stage to query whether such a structure could really have evolved as a result of tiny changes over a period of time. This same question and the argument it provokes continue to fascinate many of different persuasions who, rather than studying and analysing the diverse information and opinion that is available, prefer to use the issue to promulgate their views about the origin and significance of life. Whatever the rights and wrongs of the different arguments, none of the discussants expresses any doubt about the exquisite beauty of the eye and its importance in biology and survival!

In this book, David Williams, a veterinary surgeon with a deep interest in comparative medicine and many years' experience as an ophthalmologist, provides information and guidance about the ocular disorders of 'exotic pets'. He interprets the latter term as meaning those species that are commonly kept as companion animals but which fall outside the traditional teaching remit of the veterinary curriculum (in his words, 'non-dog-and-cat species'). His approach in the text is refreshingly personal, the prose often taking the form of familiar conversational English or expressed as a rhetorical question. This helps make this a very readable book as well as a volume that is steeped in extensive personal experience, sound clinico-pathological description and strongly evidence-based advice.

I have known Dr David Williams for many years and have always been impressed by his energy, industry and enthusiasm. These attributes have spanned the period since he worked with me as a student – and brought a new dynamism to my laboratory – to the present day, when he has evolved into a respected academic and a much appreciated teacher and mentor. His deep interest in the history of his subject, as illustrated in the introductory chapter of this book as well as his choice of images, prompts me to liken him to one of my own heroes. Jan Swammerdam (1637–1680) was a member of the Dutch school of anatomy, and, amongst many other scientific and religious pursuits, despite a traumatic period in his life, dissected and described the morphology of a whole range of vertebrate and (especially) invertebrate animals. In particular, Swammerdam performed the first comprehensive scientific studies on the anatomy of the honey bee, *Apis mellifera*, which included research on the compound and simple eyes of the species. He showed that painting over the eyes of honey bees caused them loss of sight and, using very basic microscopical equipment, he sketched the minute ocular structures that he saw, such as pigment granules and the corneal facets, those elongated crystalline cones that are typical of the species. David Williams is very much in the same mould; he shares Swammerdam's fascination with the mysteries of the natural world and he is endowed with comparable dedication to his subject and attention to detail.

*'Nanos gigantium humeris insidentes'*; those of us with a passion for the study of comparative medicine and its application to diverse species are mere dwarfs compared with the pioneers who, decades ago, investigated and marvelled at what were described by Darwin as 'endless forms most beautiful and most wonderful'. David Williams is conscious of these antecedents and in his book he pays generous tribute to those, both from the present and the past, who have helped pave the way for his many achievements.

The provision of proper veterinary attention to exotic pets is essential if these animals, which play an important part in society by providing companionship and education, are to thrive. Specialist texts are greatly needed and this volume by David Williams will admirably fill the gap as far as the ophthalmology of exotic pets is concerned. It will, I believe, not only provide advice of the highest quality but also prove fun to read and to use. I wish it well.

*John E Cooper*, DTVM FRCPath FSB CBiol FRCVS

RCVS Specialist in Veterinary Pathology
Diplomate, European College of Veterinary Pathologists
European Veterinary Specialist, Zoological Medicine

Faculty of Veterinary Medicine, University of Nairobi, Kenya
Department of Veterinary Medicine, University of Cambridge, UK
Durrell Institute of Conservation and Ecology (DICE),
The University of Kent, UK.

# Acknowledgements

To all who provided my education in exotic ophthalmology, cases to see and images to borrow: most particularly John Cooper, Elliott Jacobson, Steve Barten, Kathy Barrie, Willy Wildgoose, Peter Lee, Sheila Crispin and Graham Martin.

# Dedication

To Jennie, who puts up with me spending far too much time in the chaos of my study, and to Sam, Jack and Ross, who live with my gruesome eye images on screen and exotic eyeballs in pots, here there and everywhere!

And not forgetting God, who designed all these wonderful eyes in the first place!

# Chapter 1

# Introduction

The quite remarkable feature of eyes across vertebrate species from the axolotl to the zebra is their similarity. The basic design of the eye, the cornea, the iris, the lens, the retina all enclosed in a tough collagenous sclera, is duplicated throughout vertebrate species, as are the similar functions across the animal kingdom with light refracted to form an image on the retina where the photoreceptors transform the incident photon's energy into an electrical signal.

And yet these eyes have many differences in both their anatomy and their pathology: their appearance when normal and abnormal. Let's face it, if this were not the case there would honestly be no need for this book! From the differences in conjunctival responses to infectious organisms to the variation in vascular anatomy of the orbit in the rabbit as compared to that of the dog and cat we are more used to enucleating, it is vital to understand the variation in anatomy and physiology, in pharmacology and pathology between the eyes of fish, amphibians, reptiles, birds and mammals.

Indeed this could be replicated across body systems but not perhaps quite so dramatically as in the eye. There is a dichotomy in exotic animal veterinary medicine. On the one hand quite a substantial proportion of what we understand about the diseases of cats and dogs, their aetiopathology and their management can be extrapolated to help us deal with disease in less familiar species, be they raptors or rabbits. But on the other hand there are differences between hounds, hamsters and horned toads that make extrapolation without due care and attention potentially ineffective or even dangerous.

Hopefully this volume will aid in identifying where extrapolation from canine and feline ophthalmology can be made and where new information is necessary. We start with areas where extrapolation is possible, the first of these being the straightforward techniques of ocular examination, which may, in many cases, be transferred from conventional companion animal species. Even here though, differences exist.

Before we continue, however, it may be that this is an appropriate point to make two confessions. First some might complain that there are several areas of duplication in the text. The book is designed with the assumption that many will not read it through from cover to cover, but rather use it as a reference dipping in to specific ocular diseases in particular species. Thus several areas are necessarily somewhat duplicated to ensure that

*Ophthalmology of Exotic Pets*, First Edition. David L. Williams.
© 2012 David Williams. Published 2012 by Blackwell Publishing Ltd.

the information needed is presented in a readily accessible form. Second it might be necessary to give an apology to some for the wording of the title of this book 'Ophthalmology of Exotic Pets'. For some, it must be noted, rabbits and guinea pigs are hardly exotic species; recent evidence suggests that rabbits are the third most common species seen in small animal veterinary practice, certainly here in the United Kingdom and quite possibly elsewhere also. Nevertheless in many ways, from their teeth to their retinas, rabbits and guinea pigs are very different from cats and dogs and so they deserve inclusion in a volume detailing ophthalmic disease in what we might term non-dog-and-cat species. But that would hardly make an appropriate title for a book like this would it?! My first reason for producing a volume on this subject came when seeing how useful Sue Paterson's volume 'Skin Diseases of Exotic Pets' was [1]. Sue cleverly gathered a group of other dermatologists with special interests in different exotic species to write her book with her, but somehow I failed to galvanise others in the field of veterinary ophthalmology to produce a similar volume. I hope that those with greater expertise and experience in the fields of reptile, avian and laboratory animal ophthalmology will forgive any resulting failings in this book. Perhaps a second edition can include their contributions to the subject.

## Reference

1. Paterson S. *Skin Diseases of Exotic Pets*. Oxford: Blackwell Publishing, 2006.

# Chapter 2

# A brief history of comparative ophthalmology

While we may think that a text on exotic animal ophthalmology is a new venture, and certainly within veterinary ophthalmology this is the first volume dedicated to the subject, ophthalmologists and visual scientists have for many years considered the delights of comparative ophthalmology worth pursuing. The great Sir Stewart Duke Elder started his momentous 16 volume *System of Ophthalmology* with a glorious first volume entitled 'The Eye in Evolution', covering ocular anatomy and physiology together with visual ecology and behaviour from invertebrates through to higher mammals. But 50 years earlier the Canadian ophthalmologist Casey Albert Wood (Figure 2.1) was already publishing his remarkable overview of avian ophthalmology *The Fundus Oculi of Birds as Viewed with the Ophthalmoscope* linking his lifelong interest in ornithology with his acknowledged expertise in ophthalmology.

Wood, born in Ontario, Canada in 1856, first studied medicine in Montreal with further studies at Berlin, Vienna, Paris and London where he worked at Moorfields. He studied in Montreal under William (later Sir William) Osler and it was at this early stage that his passion for ophthalmology began. Before then however, even from childhood, his second passion, for nature study and particularly ornithology, took root. Together ophthalmology and ornithology would guide Wood through his life. Having no children, he, his wife Emma and their pet parrot John Paul toured the globe after his retirement in 1906, collecting material for his magnum opus on the appearance of the avian retina, published in 1917 (Figure 2.2). This was not just a work arising from a general interest in birds. Wood considered that the superior optics and visual capability of many birds when compared with the human eye may well lead to discoveries which would improve human vision.

But while *The Fundus Oculi of Birds* is the book for which Wood is remembered today, he was a key general ophthalmologist in North America at the end of the nineteenth century, one might even argue the key ophthalmologist. His 1896 publication implicating methyl alcohol in the etiology of toxic amblyopia was considered a classic work, and Wood was editor at various times of the Ophthalmic Record, the Annals of Ophthalmology, and the American Journal of Ophthalmology (of which he was a founder in 1884). He wrote of *A System of Ophthalmic Therapeutics* (1909), *A System of Ophthalmic Operations*

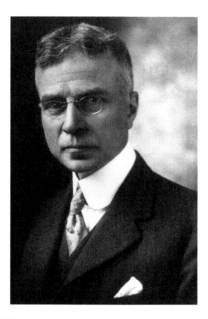

**Figure 2.1**   Casey Albert Wood.

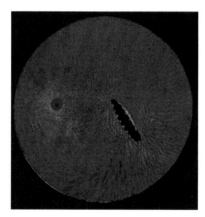

**Figure 2.2**   The tawny owl retina from *The Fundus Oculi of Birds*, 1917.

(1911), and the seventeen-volume *American Encyclopedia of Ophthalmology* (1914–1920). But more than that, Wood was fascinated by the history of ophthalmology and, of course, by comparative ophthalmology. Wood translated numerous historical ophthalmic texts from all over the world into English. A masterpiece is his translation of the earliest printed book on ophthalmology, *De Oculis Eorumque Egritudinibus et Curis*, written by the twelfth-century physician, Benvenuto Grassi, and first published in Ferrara in 1474.

For most of his working life Casey Wood was an ophthalmologist in Chicago, joining the faculty in 1899 and becoming Head of Ophthalmology in 1913, when the College of Physicians and Surgeons of Chicago became the University of Illinois College of

Medicine and holding that position until 1917. He was described as 'one of the most colorful and outstanding figures in ophthalmology at the turn of the century, not only in Chicago but nationally and internationally as well.' In 1929 Wood organized the ornithological titles at the British Museum and prepared its first catalogue describing that collection. Travelling widely in pursuit of this interest, he collected specimens in British Guiana, the Caribbean, the South Pacific, India, Ceylon, Australia and New Zealand. Wood retired from the College in 1925, spending much of his last decade at the Vatican Library in the translation of medieval European and Arabic ophthalmic manuscripts.

It has to be said that from a political perspective Wood held some views with which we might not agree – he was an ardent fascist, supporting Mussolini in the 1930s while he worked in Europe towards the end of his life, but had progressive views on the importance of animal experimentation held in balance with animal welfare. These opinions stemmed from his interest both in human medicine and also in environmental conservation, developed in his early childhood in the fields around his home in Ontario.

Another important ophthalmologist of the turn of the twentieth century with an abiding passion for comparative ophthalmology was George Lindsay Johnson (Figure 2.3). Born in 1853 and dying in 1943, Johnson was almost exactly Wood's contemporary. Interestingly, while Wood spent a formative period of his professional life in Germany, Johnson's early education occurred there although he had been born in Manchester. He was in Strasbourg in 1870 when the Prussians seized the city in a devastating episode in the Franco-Prussian war. Escaping from the beleaguered city, he spent a year on a relative's ranch in Australia before returning to his roots and studying at Owen's College in Manchester. He then undertook his undergraduate degree at Caius College in Cambridge and St Bartholomew's Hospital in London, becoming a Fellow of the Royal College of Surgeons in 1884 and taking his MD from Cambridge in 1890. His ophthalmic career

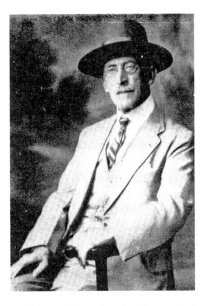

**Figure 2.3**  George Lindsay Johnson. Reproduced with permission from Elsevier.

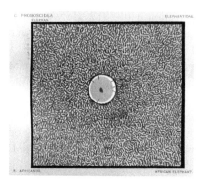

**Figure 2.4**   The fundus of the elephant from Johnson's 1902 monograph.

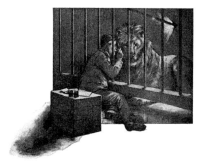

**Figure 2.5**   Arthur Head examining the fundus of a lion.

began as a registrar at the Royal Westminster Hospital in London followed by a period at the Royal Eye Hospital in Southwark, London.

During this period in London, he spent much of his spare time at the Zoological Society of London performing ophthalmic observations on a wide variety of species; this resulted in papers in the Philosophical Transactions of the Royal Society of London first on the comparative ophthalmoscopy of the mammalian eye and secondly a sequel on the eyes of reptiles and amphibians (Figure 2.4).

In this he was ably assisted by Arthur Head, ophthalmic artist of no mean distinction, as may be observed looking at his illustrations of the fundus of species from tigers to rattlesnakes (Figure 2.5). Head was also responsible for the illustrations in Wood's *The Fundus Oculi of Birds*, most of which were also undertaken in painstaking hours in the Zoological Collection at Regent's Park.

Between these two ophthalmologists of a century ago and Duke Elder stand two further key figures in the subject of comparative ocular biology. These are the French ophthalmologist, Andre Jean Francois Rochon-Duvigneaud, and the American, Gordon Walls. Rochon-Duvigneaud (Figure 2.6) will be remembered for his comment that a raptor was 'a wing guided by an eye' but had considerably wider comparative interests, documented in his book *Les Yeux et la Vision des Vertebres* of 1943 [1]. But his studies ranged far wider than merely the avian eye. Born in 1863 he studied medicine in the Faculte de Bordeaux and later in Paris writing a seminal doctoral thesis on the anatomy of the human

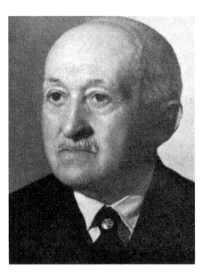

**Figure 2.6**   Andre Rochon-Duvigneaud. Reproduced with permission from Elsevier.

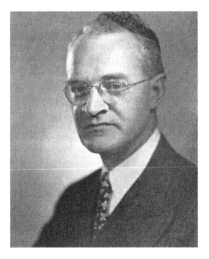

**Figure 2.7**   Gordon Walls.

iridocorneal angle in 1892. His studies took him from the human eye to a more comparative approach and, in 1926, rather in the same way Wood had done ten years earlier, he retired from clinical practice to devote his time to comparative ophthalmology. He was the first to recognise recessively inherited glaucoma with buphthalmos in the New Zealand White rabbit as far back as 1921 [2] although in human ophthalmology he is more commonly associated with the syndrome resulting from traumatic collapse of the superior orbital fissure with damage to the nerves passing through it, which bears his name [3].

Gordon Walls (Figure 2.7) was the only one of our comparative ophthalmic investigators who was not first a human ophthalmologist. He published a number of papers and monographs in comparative ophthalmology but is primarily remembered for his master-piece *The Vertebrate Eye and its Adaptive Radiation* [4] which was published a year earlier than Rochon-Duvigneaud's text. Walls was originally an engineer, moving into zoology in Harvard where he undertook work on the ultrastructure of the retina across the vertebrates. Study of the reptile eye in particular allowed him to formulate many of his ideas on the evolution of the vertebrate photoreceptor but as his magnum opus shows, his interest in development of the eye through evolution ranged across its whole anatomy and physiology, his life's work finishing with study of the intricacies of comparative colour vision on the one hand and of the evolution of ocular movement and extraocular muscle action on the other.

In the last half century and more since the deaths of Wood, Johnson, Rochon-Duvigneaud and Walls, the subject of visual ecology has become a recognised discipline, with researchers correlating visual function with behaviour of species in the wild from the visual capabilities of deep sea fish to the hunting behaviour of birds of prey. Several books on the subject are worthy of perusal. Here we add a paragraph or two on visual function in the species discussed before detailing the diseases seen in these animals. Clearly in such a limited compass detailed evaluation is not possible and thus the reader is directed to the works of Ron Douglas [5], Michael Land and Dan-Eric Nilson [6], Ivan Schwab [7] and Chris Murphy [8].

# References

1. The avian portion of the work is available online at http://www.theavianeye.com/translated.
2. Rochon-Duvigneaud A. Un cas de buphthalmie chez le lapin: etude anatomique et physi-ologique. Ann Oculist (Paris) 1921;158:401–414.
3. Rochon-Duvigneaud A. Quelques cas de paralysie de tous les nerfs orbitaires (ophthalmoplegie totale avec amaurosse en anesthésie dans le domaine de l'ophthalmique d'origine syphilitique). Archives D'ophthalmologie (Paris) 1896;16:746–760.
4. Walls GL. *The Vertebrate Eye and its Adaptive Radiation*. Bloomfield Hills, MI: The Cranbrook Institute of Science, 1942.
5. Douglas RH, Djamgoz MBA. *The Visual System of Fish*. London: Chapman and Clarke, 1990.
6. Land MF, Nilsson D-E. *Animal Eyes*. Oxford: Oxford University Press, 2002.
7. Schwab IR. From eye spots to eye shine. Br J Ophthalmol 2000;84:1214. (The first in a won-derful series of annotated cover illustrations ranging across the field of ocular evolution. Schwab's masterpiece *Evolution's Witness: How Eyes Evolved* (Oxford University Press, 2011) is a 'must-read')
8. Murphy CJ, Kern TJ, Howland HC. Refractive state, corneal curvature, accommodative range and ocular anatomy of the Asian elephant (*Elephas maximus*). Vision Research 1992;32:2013–2021. (One of a number of papers on the refractive status of a wide range of non-domestic species.)

# Chapter 3

# Common features of exotic animal ophthalmology

We will discuss the ocular anatomy and physiology of different species groups at the beginning of each chapter together with an assessment of how and what the different species actually see. Here we consider some areas which unite the different types of animal eye, before moving on to examine fish, amphibians, reptiles, birds and mammal species individually in detail.

## Ocular examination

The similarity between eyes of different species means that the basic techniques of ocular examination can be extrapolated from those of dogs and cats. The differences generally occur because of the small size of many eyes of exotic animal species, be they rodents, caged birds or reptiles.

From one perspective a direct ophthalmoscope can be used whatever the size of the globe. And yet the ease of examination and the quality of retinal image is indeed reduced with a pupil of 2 or 3 mm compared with the dilated dog or cat pupil at nearly 10 mm in diameter.

Whether used on a small rodent or a large dog, the direct ophthalmoscope can be used at 0 dioptres (D) as the cornea and lens refract the incoming light on to the retina whatever the size of the globe. Similarly using the direct ophthalmoscope at +10 D focuses light on the lens and iris and at +20 D the cornea can be seen at high magnification (Figure 3.1). It has to be said that most veterinary ophthalmologists who regularly examine rodents use the indirect technique and a +30 D lens to examine the eye [1]. But the technique one learns while training tends to stick and Dr Keith Barnett who inspired me and taught me all I know about veterinary ophthalmology always used the direct ophthalmoscope, so that is what I feel most familiar with. Professor Peter Bedford, with whom I worked later in my ophthalmic training, never seemed to pick up a direct, always using the binocular indirect for examination of the retina using the loupe lens at a distance (Figure 3.2) and the lens and cornea at a shorter distance from the eye (Figure 3.3).

Using a +30 D or even a higher dioptre lens can give a signficantly wider view of the retina than a direct ophthalmoscope but is quite a difficult technique to master. It requires

*Ophthalmology of Exotic Pets*, First Edition. David L. Williams.
© 2012 David Williams. Published 2012 by Blackwell Publishing Ltd.

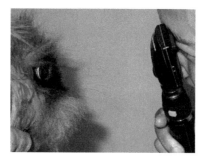

**Figure 3.1**   Using the direct ophthalmoscope to examine a rabbit eye.

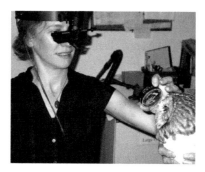

**Figure 3.2**   Using an indirect ophthalmoscope to examine the fundus of an owl eye.

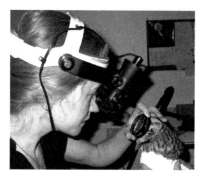

**Figure 3.3**   Using the indirect ophthalmoscope to examine the anterior segment of an owl eye.

as dilated a pupil as possible, which brings us on to another problem with a number of exotic species, that of mydriasis. A novel and useful technique recent published for rodent fundus imaging and photography, a notoriously taxing exercise, is the use of a video endoscope [2].

The small size of the eye means that the slit lamp with its high magnification is very useful in many of these species (Figure 3.4) [3]. Although, as its name suggests, this instrument is optimally used with a slit beam of light creating an optic cross-section of the ocular tissues observed, most of the time veterinary ophthalmologists use it with a full beam of light as a binocular magnifying system, especially where the small eyes of most exotic pet species are concerned.

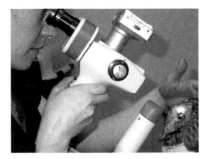

**Figure 3.4**   Using a slit lamp biomicroscope to examine the anterior segment of the eye.

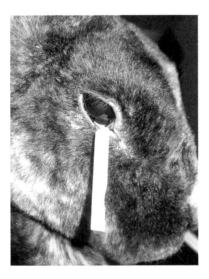

**Figure 3.5**   The Schirmer tear test used on a rabbit.

## Ancillary tests

Two key tests which should be undertaken as routine supplementation to straightforward ocular examination are the measurement of tear production and the determination of intraocular pressure. The small size of most eyes examined herein renders their tear volume similarly minute. The standard method of measuring lacrimation, the Schirmer tear test, while it can be of use in sizeable animals such as the rabbit (Figure 3.5) and larger bird species, is just too big to fit in the palpebral aperture of many smaller species, and the tear volume available to be taken up by the test strip is just too small. Here the phenol red thread test is ideal [4–7]. Held in the eye for 15 seconds (Figure 3.6) it gives a measurable reading of reddened thread by taking up a very small volume of tears. The only problems are the limited availability of the threads, their price and the paucity of normal values for many species. For some species groups we do have data, these produced in each of the following chapters. However, for all too many animals we have no values for normal animals. In such cases the normal fellow eye can be used in animals unilaterally affected, or readings can be taken on an unaffected cage-mate. A simpler test

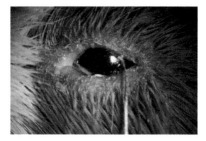

**Figure 3.6**   The phenol red thread test used on a guinea pig.

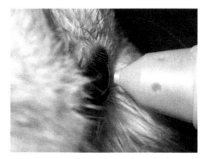

**Figure 3.7**   The Tonopen applanation tonometer used on a rabbit eye.

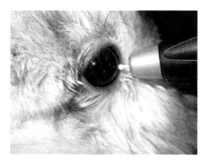

**Figure 3.8**   The Tonovet rebound tonometer used on a rabbit eye.

may be to cut the Schirmer tear test strip in half, as has been reported by Rudolph Korbel in owls; we await studies of normal tear wetting values in other species for this inexpensive and readily available test.

Measuring intraocular pressure (IOP) should be a standard test for any animal with a red eye, with glaucoma (and a raised IOP) or uveitis (with a correspondingly lower value) two important diagnoses differentiated by tonometry. Again in these small eyes the problem is that our standard test, applanation tonometry using the Tonopen (Figure 3.7), has just too big a footplate for any eye with a corneal diameter less than 5 mm. The Tonovet rebound tonometer (Figure 3.8), designed first for use in laboratory rodents [8,9], is invaluable in many small species [10]. Again we do not have much in the way of normal data, but our studies so far indicate that there is enough similarity between the

Tonovet and Tonopen values in larger eyes, to allow us to diagnose cases where IOP a measured with the Tonovet rebound tonometer is over 20 mmHg (glaucoma) or under 10 mmHg (uveitis).

## Ocular pharmacology

As will be discussed in more detail in each species group where it is relevant, mydriasis can be a significant problem in different exotic animals. The mammals have autonomically innervated iris musculature which means that parasympatholytic agents such as atropine and tropicamide are generally effective in providing pupil dilation. Having said that, rabbits and rodents with pigmented irides often show poor or slowly acting pharmacologically mediated mydriasis. Some contain atropinase [11], an enzyme that breaks down atropine, while in others the drug is bound to pigment, changing its efficacy [12].

The lack of mydriasis mediated by these muscarinic parasympatholytic agents in reptiles and birds occurs because here the muscles of the iris are not smooth muscles, autonomically innervated as in the mammals, but rather striated muscles similar to those of the limbs. Here mydriasis requires a non-depolarising muscle relaxant, such as vecuronium [13,14] or pancuronium, or indeed a depolarizing agent such as succinyl choline [15], The latter is used far less commonly as it has to be injected intracamerally, into the eye; not ideal in a bird or reptile needing mydriasis.

Another important pharmacological factor in many exotic animal species concerns the fact that with such a small globe size, and indeed a small blood volume, using the same size of eye drop that one would employ in a dog a thousand times as big as a laboratory rodent or a bird, must give a high risk of substantial systemic toxicity. Unless we use an applicator such as a Gilson pipette that can deliver a 5 µl drop rather than the normal 25–30 µl size that comes out of a standard dropper bottle, we risk such toxicity. Indeed reducing the drop volume, and thus the total drug instilled into the eye, actually increases the bioavailable drug in the eye after topical administration as was shown in a beautiful series of papers by Patton more than 30 years ago [16].

## References

1. Williams DL. Rabbit and rodent ophthalmology. Eur J Comp Anim Pract 2008;17:242–252.
2. Guyomard JL, Rosolen SG, Paques M, Delyfer MN, Simonutti M, Tessier Y, Sahel JA, Legargasson JF, Picaud S. A low-cost and simple imaging technique of the anterior and posterior segments: eye fundus, ciliary bodies, iridocorneal angle. Invest Ophthalmol Vis Sci 2008;49:5168–5174.
3. Hess HH, Newsome DA, Knapka JJ, Westney GE. Slitlamp assessment of age of onset and incidence of cataracts in pink-eyed, tan-hooded retinal dystrophic rats. Curr Eye Res 1982–1983;2:265–269.
4. Storey ES, Carboni DA, Kearney MT, Tully TN. Use of phenol red thread tests to evaluate tear production in clinically normal Amazon parrots and comparison with Schirmer tear test findings. J Am Vet Med Assoc 2009;235:1181–1187.
5. Trost K, Skalicky M, Nell B. Schirmer tear test, phenol red thread tear test, eye blink frequency and corneal sensitivity in the guinea pig. Vet Ophthalmol 2007;10:143–146.

6. Holt E, Rosenthal K, Shofer FS. The phenol red thread tear test in large Psittaciformes. Vet Ophthalmol 2006;9:109–113.
7. Biricik HS, Oğuz H, Sindak N, Gürkan T, Hayat A. Evaluation of the Schirmer and phenol red thread tests for measuring tear secretion in rabbits. Vet Rec 2005;156:485–487.
8. Kontiola AI, Goldblum D, Mittag T, Danias J. The induction/impact tonometer: a new instrument to measure intraocular pressure in the rat. Exp Eye Res 2001;73:781–785.
9. Danias J, Kontiola AI, Filippopoulos T, Mittag T. Method for the noninvasive measurement of intraocular pressure in mice. Invest Ophthalmol Vis Sci 2003;44:1138–1141.
10. Jeong MB, Kim YJ, Yi NY, Park SA, Kim WT, Kim SE, Chae JM, Kim JT, Lee H, Seo KM. Comparison of the rebound tonometer (TonoVet) with the applanation tonometer (TonoPen XL) in normal Eurasian Eagle owls (*Bubo bubo*). Vet Ophthalmol 2007;10:376–379.
11. Salazar M, Patil PN. An explanation for the long duration of mydriatic effect of atropine in eye. Invest Ophthalmol 1976;15:671–673.
12. Salazar M, Shimada K, Patil PN. Iris pigmentation and atropine mydriasis. J Pharmacol Exp Ther 1976;197:79–88.
13. Mikaelian I, Paillet I, Williams D. Comparative use of various mydriatic drugs in kestrels (*Falco tinnunculus*). Am J Vet Res 1994;55:270–272.
14. Ramer JC, Paul-Murphy J, Brunson D, Murphy CJ. Effects of mydriatic agents in cockatoos, African gray parrots, and blue-fronted Amazon parrots. J Am Vet Med Assoc 1996;208:227–230.
15. Verschueren CP, Lumeij JT. Mydriasis in pigeons (*Columbia livia domestica*) with d-tubocurarine: topical instillation versus intracameral injection. J Vet Pharmacol Ther 1991;14:206–208.
16. Patton TF. Pharmacokinetic evidence for improved ophthalmic drug delivery by reduction of instilled volume. J Pharm Sci 1977;66:1058–1059.

# Chapter 4

# The rabbit eye

## Introduction

Ocular diseases have commonly been diagnosed in the rabbit for many years [1], particularly in laboratory strains where infectious conditions were common and important [2], but recently ophthalmic disease has been seen more and more in pet animals also. Thus while what we might call the basic sciences of the rabbit eye have been known for decades, it is only in the past few years that rabbit ophthalmology as a discipline with a proper diagnostic and therapeutic foundation has taken off. And thus there are still many areas, from dacryocystitis to cataract extraction, where we still have a long way to go before eye disease in rabbits is managed as adequately as it is in dogs and cats.

While there are several reports of ocular disease in the rabbit, we do not currently have a study of the prevalence of ocular disease in this species. In an attempt to mirror the study we have conducted in 1000 guinea pigs (see Chapter 5) we have just finished a study documenting eye disease in 1000 pet rabbits and hope to analyse our findings and publish in the peer-reviewed literature in the near future. Preliminary findings note that 26% of rabbits were found to have ocular lesions with 17% having some degree of lens opacification, 3.5% with dacryocystitis and 2.5% with corneal lesions from chronic scarring to frank ulceration. Such figures vary from those seen in laboratory animals [3] and from those in the referral hospital population [4], but we hope that they are more representative of the disease prevalence in the normal pet population, at least in the United Kingdom.

## Anatomy and physiology of the rabbit eye

Given the widespread use of the rabbit as an experimental animal model for ocular disease it might be thought surprising that we only have one detailed text describing its ocular anatomy and physiology, and that from Prince back in 1954 [5]! In some ways the rabbit eye is similar to ours and that of domestic animals in its general layout, but in others, particularly with regard to its retinal organisation, it is quite different.

*Ophthalmology of Exotic Pets*, First Edition. David L. Williams.
© 2012 David Williams. Published 2012 by Blackwell Publishing Ltd.

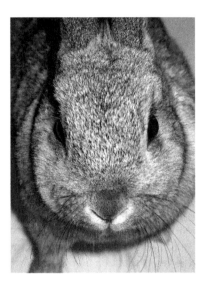

**Figure 4.1**   The lateral placement of the rabbit eye with substantial exposure even in the normal animal.

The eyes are placed very prominently and laterally (Figure 4.1) to allow the wide visual fields experienced by the wild rabbit which can see almost the entirety of its environment from far anteriorly to right behind its head; below we will discuss further where this might not be true in pet rabbits. Interestingly this very lateral placement has implications for the inflammatory mechanisms within the eye quite as much as the neurobiology of vision. As noted in a wonderful paper by Laslo Bitto, this prominence means that the eye can quite readily be damaged [6]. The intraocular inflammatory cascade following injury is thus quite profound and rapid with production of fibrinous secondary aqueous after loss of fluid from the eye in a much more substantial manner than is the case for the human eye, where our brow and totally enclosed bony orbit protects the globe from injury. Such differences are important to note either when considering the rabbit as an experimental model for intraocular inflammatory disease or when assessing its response to therapeutic intraocular surgery.

The lagormorph nasolacrimal system is unique with one nasolacrimal punctum and a nasolacrimal duct which takes a tortuous route to the nasal ostium with two sharp diversions and narrowings and an anatomy which takes the duct close to the molar and incisor tooth roots; this is discussed further under dacryocystitis.

The rabbit has a circular pupil, and a heavily pigmented iris in pigmented species (Figure 4.2), with complex vascular anatomy as recently investigated through corrosion casts [7]. The vasculature of the merangiotic lagomorph fundus is unlike that of any other mammal to this author's knowledge, in that the vessels extend from the optic disc with myelinated nerve fibres horizontally (Figures 4.3 and 4.4), allowing the visual streak, lying parallel and inferior to the retinal vessels, to be supplied solely through the choroidal vessel network [8].

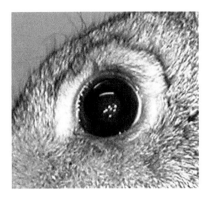

**Figure 4.2** The rabbit pupil.

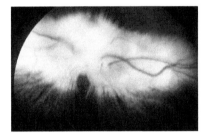

**Figure 4.3** Optic nerve head in a pigmented rabbit.

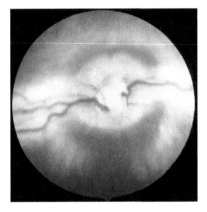

**Figure 4.4** Optic nerve head in an albino rabbit.

Another important vascular peculiarity in the lagomorph eye is the sizeable retrobulbar venous plexus (Figure 4.5) [9]. As we will see this has important implications in exophthalmos and enucleation, but the reason for this vascular arrangement, also seen to a lesser degree in smaller rodent species, remains unclear. The other orbital contents of note are the orbital glands which can make an unwelcome entrance during gland

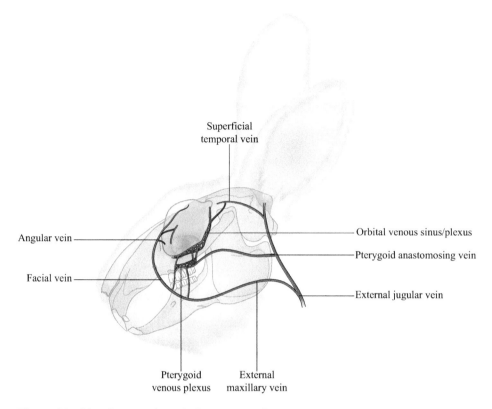

**Figure 4.5**   Line diagram of retrobulbar venous plexus.

displacement (see below) but otherwise take up a significant portion of the retrobulbar space (Figure 4.6).

## What do rabbits see?

As a prey species the rabbit has vision concentrating on the horizon with the ability to concentrate on this narrow band of visual information for almost 360 degrees of circumference (Figure 4.7). We cannot, of course, have much of an idea of what this sort of vision 'looks' like to the rabbit in the same way we cannot understand what the psychology of a prey species 'feels' like. We will encounter this problem again and again as we ask what other species' vision 'looks' like to them. The neurophysiological and electroretinographic reports we will allude to tell us something as do the visual field studies of researchers such as Martin in the avian sphere, but in essence the fact that we can know little of the sensory lives of other species is a philosophical, quite as much as a physiological or psychological one.

  As we noted above, the classic view is that rabbits can see both in front and behind them. While this is certainly true of a slim wild animal or pet breed such as a Netherland

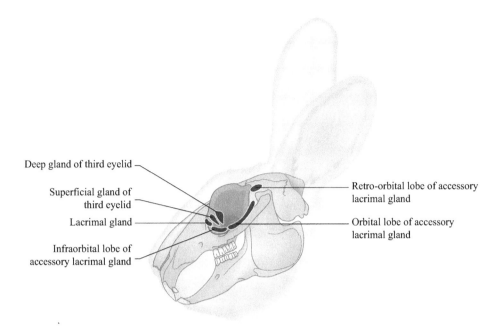

Deep gland of third eyelid

Superficial gland of
third eyelid

Lacrimal gland

Infraorbital lobe of
accessory lacrimal gland

Retro-orbital lobe of accessory
lacrimal gland

Orbital lobe of accessory
lacrimal gland

**Figure 4.6**   Line diagram of orbital glands.

dwarf, simple observation of a rather overweight lop shows that this is not always the case! Preliminary investigations similar to those of avian visual fields reported by Martin, show the variation in rabbit visual fields between different individuals (Figure 4.7) and with the head in different positions. Any rabbit with its head held up in an alert position, will indeed be able to see 360 degrees with binocular fields anetriorly, posteriorly and dorsally. But a rotund lop-eared animal in a sedentary position has very much reduced visual fields.

Concerning the eye itself, the horizontal arrangement of myelinated nerve fibres allows a long horizontal visual streak, potentially allowing the rabbit to pay high-grade attention to the horizon, and overhead presumably to detect approaching predators. The refraction of the rabbit eye has been determined as almost emmetropic at 0.5 D by electrophysio-logical means [10], although there is some debate over measurement by retinoscopy. De Graauw and Van Hof reported frontal myopia, whereby the rabbit is short-sighted when using its binocular vision anteriorly but emmetropic (normally sighted) or slightly hyper-meytropic (long-sighted) when looking laterally [11,12]. Other workers [13] could not repeat these findings and concluded that De Graauw and Van Hof's off-axis retinopscopy was inaccurate.

Determination of contrast sensitivity in Pak's report [10] achieved through meas-urement of pattern-evoked cortical potentials, suggested that the rabbit has a highest response at 0.3 cycles per degree with an upper cut-off frequency of 3 cycles per degree, giving a visual acuity of 10 minutes of arc, corresponding to a Snellen acuity of 20/200. Behavioural measurement of grating acuity with rabbits choosing a horizontal or vertical grating to obtain a food reward, demonstrated an acuity of between 1.6 and

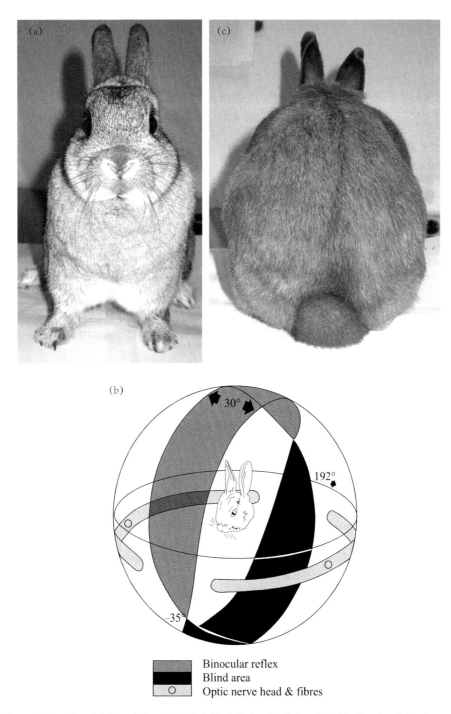

**Figure 4.7**  Visual fields of the rabbit. (a) Alert Netherland dwarf rabbit showing lateral eye placement with panoramic visual fields. (b) Diagrammatic representation of visual fields in rabbit (reproduced from Hughes A. A schematic eye for the rabbit. *Vision Research* 1972;12(1):123–38 with permission from Elsevier.). (c) Resting obese English rabbit showing lack of panoramic visual fields.

2.5 cycles/degree with different rabbits having varying acuities [14]. They all lie within the range noted by Van Hof in his 1967 paper which estimated acuity at between 1.5 and 2.7 cycles/degree. But there is more to seeing than that measured by assessment of visual acuity by Snellen charts or sinusoidal gratings. The rabbit's visual system has evolved to detect motion, and thus local edge detector ganglion cells in the retina probably allow a significantly better detection of edge and motion than this low reported visual acuity suggests [15].

As one might expect from an herbivore, detailed trichromatic color vision is not required. Indeed only 5% of the rabbit's photoreceptors are cones [16]. The two populations have maximal absorption at wavelengths of 425 nm and 520 nm corresponding to greatest sensitivity to blue and green respectively [17,18]. In the visual streak the cone density is around 13 000/mm$^2$ while in the rest of the retina it is as low as 7500/mm$^2$. Interestingly below the visual streak is a second streak containing a high proportion of blue-sensitive cones at a density of around 11 000/mm$^2$. Given that the majority of predators of the rabbit are birds, the ability to see a shape against blue in the superior visual field might seem only reasonable, while the ventral visual field is more green-sensitive.

# Adnexal disease

## Nasolacrimal disease

We start our discussion of ocular disorders with epiphora and dacryocystitis, not necessarily following the anatomical scheme we will with other species, but because of the frequency with which it is seen in the pet rabbit population, the severity of its presentation in many cases and the difficultie in its treatment [4,19,20]. Our preliminary results show a prevalence of 3.5% for dacryocystitis in the normal rabbit population. This is higher than that reported in the laboratory rabbit population [4] although those were young animals and the mean age for rabbits with the condition in our study was 5.4 years of age. Our figure is lower than that in a referral hospital population studied by Burling and colleagues [4] but hopefully presents a more normal range of cases than those referred for specialist treatment.

As noted above the rabbit nasolacrimal duct has a tortuous passage from the single ventral nasolacrimal punctum, narrowing as it passes through from the lacrimal to the frontal bones and then passing perilously close to the molar tooth roots and across the incisor tooth root before exiting in the nasal mucosa near the external nares (Figures 4.8 and 4.9) [21,22]. Thus elongation of incisor roots will obstruct nasolacrimal drainage causing epiphora, while molar tooth root abscesses will extend to involve the nasolacrimal duct with long-standing purulent dacryocystitis as a common sequel.

## Epiphora

### Clinical signs

A sizeable number of pet rabbits have epiphora as an almost normal finding with a somewhat moist periorbital region and sometimes mild conjunctivitis [23]. In a number

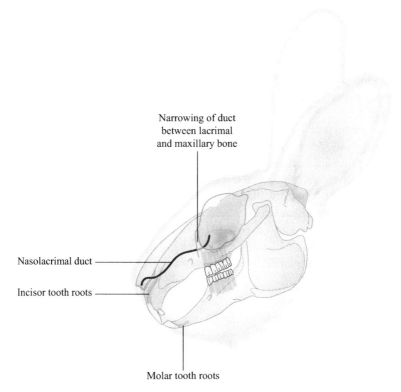

Narrowing of duct
between lacrimal
and maxillary bone

Nasolacrimal duct

Incisor tooth roots

Molar tooth roots

**Figure 4.8**   Line diagram of nasolacrimal duct.

this progresses to a severe overflow of tears yielding an excoriating facial dermatitis (Figure 4.10). The tears may be clear and watery or sometimes a whiter fluid. This is probably coloured by calcium salts rather than being exudative as with dacryocystitis (see below), where cytology will show a neutrophil population and bacteriological culture will yield a growth of organisms not generally seen in straightforward epiphora.

### Aetiopathogenesis

The close apposition of the nasolacrimal duct to the molar and incisor tooth roots (Figure 4.8) means that while the molar tooth root abscesses are the main cause of dacryocystitis, epiphora alone usually results from overgrowth of the incisor tooth root which, as it curls round ventrally, blocks the nasolacrimal duct, as shown by dacryocystorhinography of the area (Figure 4.11). There is no infection here, just a physical occlusion of the duct.

### Clinical management

Diagnostic steps in epiphora include radiography of the maxilla, important to document the involvement of dental abnormalities, and possibly also cytology and bacteriology of

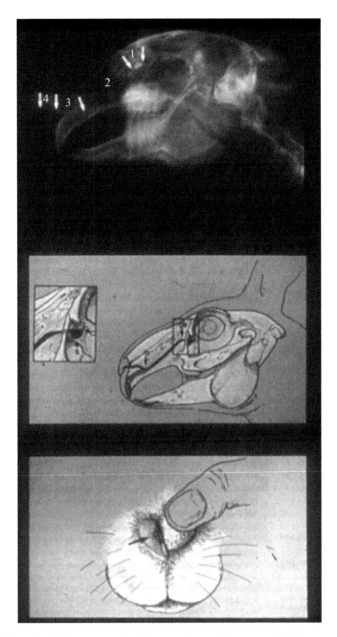

**Figure 4.9** Normal rabbit dacryocystorhinogram (top) with anatomical diagram showing association with dental roots (middle) and distal orifice (bottom). (From Burling *et al.* 1991 [4] with permission.)

tear fluid, although where this is clear in nature, an inflammatory cell picture cytologically and a meaningful bacteriological culture result are unlikely.

Flushing through the duct can be beneficial if a mucus plug is obstructing the duct. As noted above the nasolacrimal punctum of the rabbit is single and can best be cannulated by an upward pressure on the lower lid (Figure 4.12) which forces the punctum

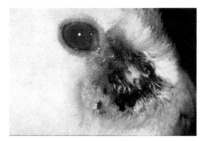

**Figure 4.10** Excoriated facial dermatitis in severe epiphora. (Reproduced with permission from Sheila Crispin.)

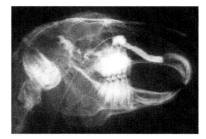

**Figure 4.11** Dacryocytorhinography of occluded nasolacrimal duct.

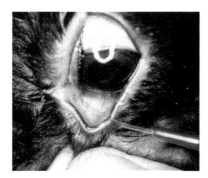

**Figure 4.12** Opening the nasolacrimal punctum.

to open with its two lips 'pouting' ready for the insertion of a narrow-gauge (23–25G) cannula. With epiphora alone this is not difficult, since the proliferative conjunctivitis (Figure 4.13) often seen in dacryocystitis (see below), which can make nasolacrimal intubation difficult, is not present. Cannulation is difficult in such circumstances and often requires the production of a new punctum through the proliferative tissue (Figure 4.14). If cannulation of the proximal punctum is impossible the distal punctum may be approached through the external nares (Figure 4.15). Mobilisation of pus by flushing in this manner will facilitate canulation of the upper punctum to allow complete flushing of the nasolacrimal duct.

Questions arise between veterinarians regarding what fluid to use for irrigation of the duct. In dacryocystitis antibiotics and anti-inflammatory agents may be worthwhile,

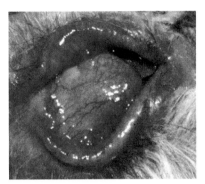

**Figure 4.13**   Proliferative conjunctivitis.

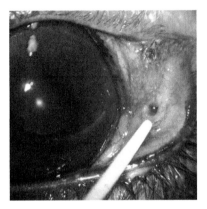

**Figure 4.14**   Cannulating the punctum in the face of severe proliferative conjunctivitis.

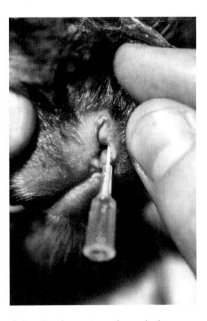

**Figure 4.15**   Cannulation of the distal punctum through the nares.

but in straightforward epiphora sterile saline is likely to be efficacious at least for a period.

## Dacryocystitis

### Clinical signs

Purulent discharge from the nasolacrimal cannaliculus is the cardinal sign of dacryocystitis but this may vary from a watery white fluid, not dissimilar to that sometimes seen in epiphora but merely more profuse (Figure 4.16), to a thick creamy white discharge, this being the more commonly seen appearance (Figure 4.17). Upward pressure with a finger on the lower eyelid will expel a bead of pus from the nasolacrimal punctum even in early cases and is a sure sign that there is inflammation and infection down the nasolacrimal duct rather than merely in the conjunctival sac. When the discharge is particularly dense it can result in an area of corneal oedema or a frank corneal ulcer in the tissue adjacent to the duct opening (Figure 4.18). Periocular swelling can be marked in some cases and in these cure is unlikely (Figure 4.19).

### Aetiopathogenesis

As noted above with epiphora, the tortuous route of the nasolacrimal duct and its proximity to the molar and incisor tooth roots means that the nasolacrimal duct is highly

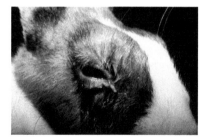

**Figure 4.16**  A wet mucopurulent discharge characteristic of early dacryocystitis.

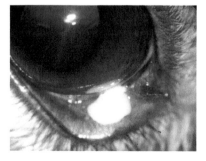

**Figure 4.17**  White discharge from nasolacrimal punctum.

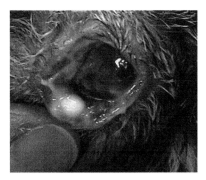

**Figure 4.18** Thick creamy white discharge with associated corneal pathology.

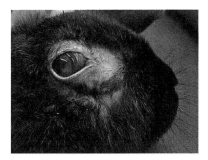

**Figure 4.19** Swelling around nasolacrimal sac.

prone to occlusion and to dilation with inflammation. The formation of dilated sacs or frank rupture of the duct next to a tooth root abscess leads to the profuse continuous purulent discharge seen. The underlying pathology of the bone of the maxilla leading to this change is associated with dietary calcium deficiency as documented in detail by Frances Harcourt-Brown whose seminal work has demonstrated the nutritional and endocrine aetiopathogenesis of this condition [24–26].

## Clinical management

Primary diagnosis of dacryocystitis is generally simple given the pathognomonic signs of purulent discharge, but determining the underlying pathology can be much more taxing. Dacryocystorhinography can be very helpful in revealing the exact location of the duct occlusion and inflammation. Injection of around 0.2 ml of a non-ionic contrast agent followed by lateral and dorsoventral radiographs shows the nasolacrimal duct, its pathology and its association with dental structures, when compared with plain radiographs taken before the contrast is used.

As noted above, long-term cure of this condition is difficult and management may be the only viable option. Topical antibiotic administration on its own is not particularly efficacious given that the duct is already blocked with purulent material. Single flushing of the duct after cannulation followed by frequent administration of topical antibiotics can have a short-term benefit but is rarely a method to control the problem in the long term. In the UK fusidic acid as Fucithalmic Vet is as licensed preparation and might be effective against staphylococcal disease but not at all against *Pasteurella*, a Gram-negative organism. In addition its viscous vehicle base, while having excellent effects in increasing drug residence time in the conjunctival sac, reduces the likelihood of it reaching deep into the nasolacrimal duct. This problem with any case of dacryocystitis whatever the species means that irrigation is a much better option than merely topical antibiosis.

Regular flushing of the duct, either with sterile saline or with antibiotics such as gentamicin or enrofloxacin, is advised by some although in some stressed animals this frequent treatment (as regular as daily for 2 weeks then every other day for a further month in some hands) may be more comprising to the rabbit's welfare than is the condition itself.

A short course of systemic antibiotic can produce a remarkably good result. Here oral azithromycin seems particularly beneficial; in this species particularly one must be very careful about enterotoxaemia from oral antibiosis, although azithromycin does not appear to have this side effect. In this author's experience 2 weeks' course of this in a paediatric elixir can have beneficial results lasting 2 or more months before another course is required. Another option is longer-term oral antibiosis. Enrofloxacin in drinking water can control the condition and surprisingly does not seem to have enterotoxaemic effects nor generate resistant strains as long as drinking water is kept with a drug dose of 5 mg/kg.

### Conjunctivitis

#### Clinical signs

Conjunctivitis in the rabbit may be very similar to inflammation of that tissue in other species. Hyperaemia is regularly associated with a proliferation of lymphoid nodules within the conjunctiva giving it a verrucose appearance with chronicity (Figure 4.13). There can be some discharge although a profuse exudate should always ring alarm bells with regard to dacryocystitis.

#### Aetiopathogenesis

All too frequently conjunctival hyperaemia, proliferation and discharge are signs of early dacryocystitis, but conjunctivitis can occur on its own from infection or from an irritative focus. This could be a single agent, such as a hay awn in the inferior conjunctival sac, or a more diffuse cause, such as a generally dusty hutch environment or a carpet shampoo used where a house rabbit resides. The difficulty in interpreting the results of a bacteriological sample can revolve around the fact that many bacteria can be normal, we might even say commensal, organisms. Even bacteria clearly recognised as pathogens in other species, such as *Pasteurella and staphylococci*, can be found in the normal rabbit nasal turbinates, and thus also conjunctiva, without causing any pathology [27]. But this is not to say that they can be ignored – in the wrong situation, and especially in an animal where the immune system is impaired, these organisms can cause significant problems. Conjunctivitis can be a manifestation of systemic infection [28], and although this is less likely than localised disease, it goes without saying that the approach to ocular infection should always involve clinical assessment of the whole animal.

## Clinical management

A key element in the history taking in cases of conjunctivitis should involve questioning the environment in which the rabbit lives.

A Schirmer tear test should be performed early in the ocular examination; while keratoconjunctivitis sicca is rare in rabbits it must be ruled out [29]. Interestingly, different breeds of rabbit have very different normal ranges of STT, emphasising the importance of comparing the patient with an unaffected cage or hutch-mate. A rabbit with an irritative conjunctivitis would be expected to have an increased tear production, so a low result compared with that of a cage-mate of the same breed for instance, should make one suspicious. Note that use of oral trimethoprim antibiotics has been shown in one recent report to reduce tear production, although the animals studied only showed a statistically significant reduction in STT after 14 days and the experiment was not extended to assess if clinical KCS occured after more prolonged drug use or whether tear production normalised on cessation of treatment [30].

Treatment of conjunctivitis where a profuse growth of a specific organism has been found should clearly be directed against that pathogen after culture and sensitivity [31]. In cases where financial constraints preclude such a full investigation, a broad-spectrum agent such as tetracycline or chloramphenicol is to be recommended. Treatment of staphylococcal conjunctivitis by production of an autologous vaccine has been reported [32] but this approach is unlikely to be widely applicable.

## Conjunctival overgrowth

### Clinical signs

This unusual condition, unique to rabbits, is readily recognised as a ring of conjunctiva growing over the cornea inwardly from the limbus (Figures 4.20, 4.21) [33–35]. The conjunctiva appears normal and not inflamed in most cases and the rest of the eye appears unremarkable [36]. The animal can see through the aperture in the central cornea where the conjunctival annulus is relatively narrow, although in some cases only a small window of cornea not covered by conjunctiva remains in the centre of the ocular surface. The key feature differentiating this from keratitis is that the conjunctiva is not adherent to the cornea.

### Aetiopathogenesis

The cause of this condition is unknown. While it has been called pseudopterygium, this is misleading since a pterygium is a fibrovascular lesion arising from the limbus in man but within the superficial cornea, while conjunctival overgrowth, also termed by some

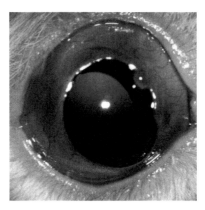

**Figure 4.20**   Mild conjunctival overgrowth in a rabbit.

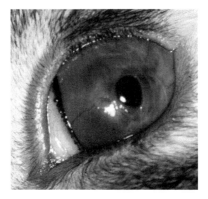

**Figure 4.21**   Marked conjunctival overgrowth in a rabbit.

conjunctival centripetalisation or epicorneal membrane [37], as noted above, is not associated with the cornea other than to lie over it.

## Clinical management

Initially veterinary ophthalmologists removed this ring of tissue by sharp dissection at
the limbus, but it was found that the tissue regrew relatively rapidly. Some reported
resection of the conjunctiva followed by application of topical cyclosporine ointment,
which appeared to prevent regrowth while it was applied. A more permanent solution is
to divide the annulus of tissue radially and then suture the conjunctiva back to the episclera so that further tissue growth does not cover the cornea (Figure 4.22) [38].

## Blepharitis

### Clinical signs

Sometimes as a part of dacryocystitis but often on its own, eyelid inflammation can
be a significant problem in rabbits. The lids become swollen and hyperaemic, losing

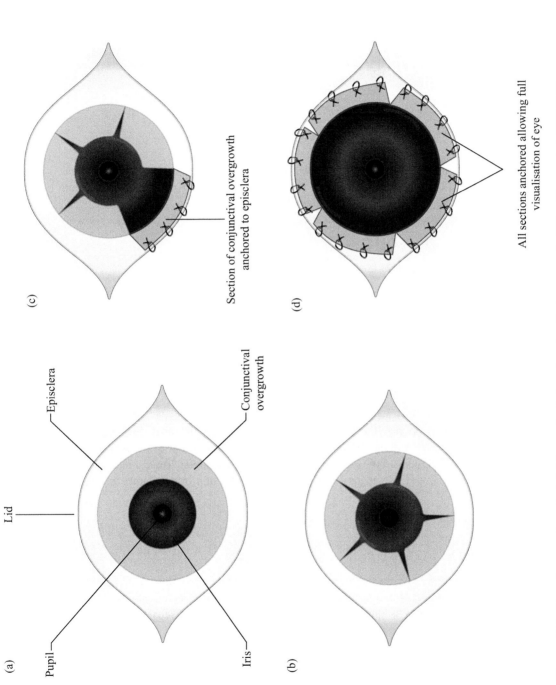

(a)

Lid

Episclera

Pupil

Iris

Conjunctival overgrowth

(b)

(c)

Section of conjunctival overgrowth anchored to episclera

(d)

All sections anchored allowing full visualisation of eye

**Figure 4.22** Line diagram of surgical division and suturing of conjunctival overgrowth. (After Allgoer *et al.* 2008 [28].)

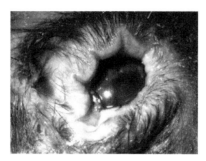

**Figure 4.23**  Blepharitis in a rabbit.

their natural apposition with the cornea (Figure 4.23), with resulting pathological changes in the ocular surface. Sometimes there is discharge associated with the condition but this may be linked with the resulting conjunctivitis and not the blepharitis itself, given that cases can be seen without the sort of discharge seen in conjunctivitis with dacryocystitis.

### Aetiopathogenesis

Blepharitis is not directly associated with specific infection, but many consider that it is associated with an allergic immune reaction to staphylococcal antigen [39]. The evidence for this may not be particularly strong in individual cases, but here one might see a similarity with juvenile pyoderma in the dog which for all the world appears to be an infectious disease but resolves not with antibiotics but with oral steroids.

### Clinical management

In this author's experience hot water compresses are probably the most efficacious treatment to reduce the swelling and improve the degree of apposition of the lids with the corneal surface to reduce both exposure keratitis and excoriation. Topical and systemic antibiosis may be valuable as may systemic non-steroidal anti-inflammatory treatment.

## Myxomatosis

### Clinical signs

This tragic viral disease results in blepharitis and conjunctivitis with a profuse purulent discharge (Figure 4.24) as a prelude to death in infected unvaccinated rabbits. The case in vaccinated animals is quite different without the purulent discharge but with the development of myxomatous masses on the lid (Figure 4.25).

### Aetiopathogenesis

The myxoma virus which causes myxomatosis is a poxvirus and as such has a large DNA genome which allows it to hijack genes from mammalian hosts. Such genes, such as

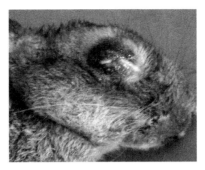

**Figure 4.24**   Myxomatosis in a wild rabbit with profuse discharge.

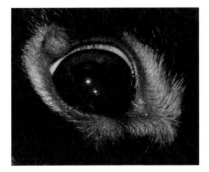

**Figure 4.25**   Myxoma development on lids of vaccinated rabbit with myxomatosis.

those for the major histocompatability complex (MHC) and cytokine homologues, allow the virus to counteract the host's immune system, preventing presentation of its antigens to host T cells and reducing the antiviral effects of T cells by competing with their own cytokines [40]. This explains the prevalence of secondary infections in affected animals, the rapid undefeated spread of the virus in the individual and their rapid demise. Quite why the pathology is particularly focused on the mucocutaneous junctions of the lid and the genitalia is, to this author at least, unclear.

### Clinical management

The preferred option in unvaccinated cases, at least in this author's opinion, is euthanasia. Although some have suggested that courses of alpha-interferon may be effective this has not be found to be the case in unvaccinated animals in this author's experience. In vaccinated animals there is rarely need for treatment, given that the only ocular signs are periocular myxomas. If tumours at the lid margin cause corneal irritation, these could be removed with a simple wedge resection, ensuring a good surgical margin is taken (perhaps 1–2 mm given the good demarcation of these neoplasms, their relatively non-aggressive local behaviour and the small aperture of the rabbit eyelid).

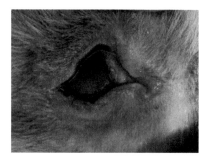

**Figure 4.26**   Entropion in a rabbit.

## Entropion

### Clinical signs

As with entropion in dogs, lid in-turning is generally seen in young rabbits, but this is relatively rare and infrequently reported. Lid in-turning is evident from close inspection, but by the time it is presented there is often corneal damage present (Figure 4.26). It can be difficult to evaluate whether the entropion is secondary to ocular irritation or whether the irritation from corneal pathology was caused by the entropion and subsequent trichiasis with eyelid hairs abrading the cornea.

### Aetiopathogenesis

Why some rabbits should be affected by entropion is unclear. There does not appear to be a particularly inherited tendency in specific rabbit strains but several animals within a litter can be affected. In certain cases the history clearly shows that an ocular surface irritative focus, such as a corneal ulcer, has provoked the entropion.

### Clinical management

A standard Hotz–Celsus procedure can be undertaken on affected rabbits, but rather in the same way that young puppies often need tacking procedures before a definitive surgical rectification, rabbit kits can require urgent action early in life to protect the corneal surface from irritation and this may be before a permanent surgical correction is possible. Temporary tacking sutures with 4/0 to 6/0 vicryl in a vertical mattress arrangement can be effective.

## Nictitans gland prolapse

### Clinical signs

In the same way as is seen in the dog, the orbital glands of the rabbit can prolapse to give the appearance of 'cherry eye' (Figure 4.27) [41,42]. The difference with the rabbit

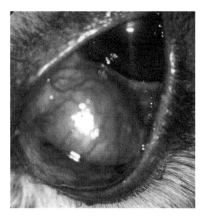

**Figure 4.27** Prolapsed Harderian gland in a rabbit.

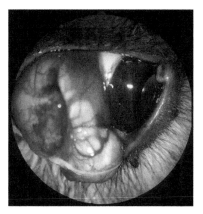

**Figure 4.28** Prolapsed Harderian and nictitans glands in a rabbit.

is that, as noted above, there are several orbital glands, one or all of which can prolapse (Figure 4.28). Thus the condition can look merely like a small well demarcated, round, pink to red mass in the medial canthus, or a rather more alarming protrusion of several different types of tissue, manifesting appearance of the deep and superficial glands of the third eyelid, the Harderian gland and the deep orbital gland, though to see all four is unusual.

## Aetiopathogenesis

Quite why gland prolapse occurs in dogs is unclear and the same is true in rabbits. It may be that a conjunctival trauma initiates the protrusion of these orbital glands or there may possibly be an anomaly in the connective tissue which normally holds them in place.

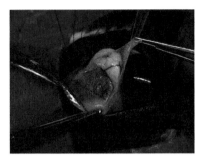

**Figure 4.29**   Repairing prolapsed gland with pocket technique.

### *Clinical management*

Some would suggest that the gland, if only one is involved, can be left prolapsed, yet experience shows, as with the case in dogs, that a protruding gland gradually becomes inflamed and enlarged – it is better replaced earlier rather than later. One might ask if the gland could be removed. In dogs we know that the nictitans gland produces around a third of the tear film. We have no such evidence for tear production in the rabbit, but one might say that as God put them there, they must have a purpose! Another reason for replacing them rather than performing gland removal is that the latter risks damaging the retrobulbar venous plexus, with potentially catastrophic haemorrhagic consequences. In the author's experience use of Dr Rhea Morgan's pocket technique [43] for such glands in the rabbit is relatively easy and successful (Figure 4.29); attempting to fix the glands to the orbital rim using the technique described by Dr Renee Kaswan [44] would be difficult since, while the superficial gland of the nictitating membrane might be suitable for such a technique, the other glands are either too friable or to multilobulated to allow a single suture to hold them in place.

### *Microphthalmos*

### *Clinical signs*

Congenital abnormalities in globe size can occur in any species but seem to be rarely reported in the rabbit. Microphthalmos can occur through genetic or nutritional agency. While no treatment is possible, attempts to define the aetiology are important to prevent future cases of the condition [45].

## Diseases of the orbit

### *Exophthalmos*

Protrusion of the globe from the orbit is relatively common in rabbits for a number of reasons (Figures 4.30 and 4.31). The eye is relatively prominent so a space-occupying

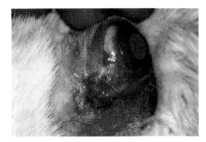

**Figure 4.30** Exophthalmos in rabbit.

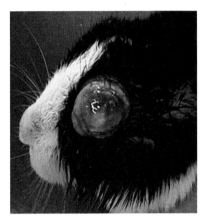

**Figure 4.31** Exophthalmos in rabbit.

lesion in the orbit, be it infectious, neoplastic, parasitic or vascular, will readily manifest as an exophthalmic globe. Determination of the reason for globe protrusion is often best achieved by cranial radiography and orbital ultrasonography, although other imaging techniques can be valuable if more expensive, and sometimes clinical judgement on its own can be sufficient to yield a diagnostic result.

## Orbital abscessation

### Clinical signs

The most common cause of exophthalmos, and thus the first diagnosis to rule out, is that of an orbital abscess from a molar tooth root. These can occur rapidly and give severe exophthalmos often with exposure keratitis and strabismus. Radiography demonstrating a tooth root abscess impinging on the orbital contents is diagnostic, although imaging techniques such as magnetic resonance imaging (MRI) or computed tomography (CT) can delineate the lesion more precisely (Figure 4.32). Examination of the dentition is mandatory and a haemogram will confirm an inflammatory focus, though clearly not define its position.

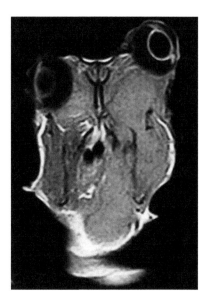

**Figure 4.32**   MRI scan of rabbit in Figure 4.31 showing large tooth root abscess.

### Aetiopathogenesis

The vast majority of orbital abscesses in rabbits are associated with molar tooth root problems and as such cure is very difficult to achieve. Other reports of lesions giving rise to exophthalmos include those of parasitic cysts [46] and neoplasms [47] in the orbit.

### Clinical management

Enucleation together with exenteration of infected orbital contents can ameliorate signs, though on its own this is only a temporary solution. In all too many cases even the most aggressive enucleation eventually fails as remaining bacteria proliferate and the orbital abscess recurs, eventually breaking through the enucleation incision. The use of antibiotic-impregnated beads in the orbit can improve the prognosis which is grave in the majority of cases. Manuka honey in the enucleated or exenterated orbit has been suggested as a worthwhile therapeutic option and in an admittedly small number of cases to date we have found this very useful in sterilising open orbits after exenteration and in promoting a granulation tissue response [48].

### Retrobulbar venous plexus engorgement

### Clinical signs

The unusual appearance of a rabbit which becomes bilaterally exophthalmic when stressed is a pathognomonic sign of retrobulbar venous plexus engorgement (Figure 4.33) [49,50]. The stressor sufficient to cause a rise in blood pressure sufficient to overfill the

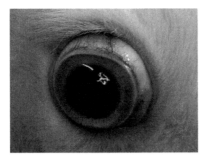

**Figure 4.33** Periodic exophthalmos in rabbit with thymoma.

venous plexus when vascular drainage is compromised can be as mild as gentle stroking. Perhaps this is enough to alert us to the parless state of this prey species in our care even when we think we are calming it down!

### Aetiopathogenesis

Most of the cases reported with this condition have been affected by a cranial thoracic space-occupying lesion such as a thymoma. The neoplasm enwraps the jugular veins restricting venous return from the head. With mildly increased arterial blood pressure during a stressful period it is assumed (although to the author's knowledge nobody has measured this parameter in these animals during such stressing) that the increased arterial filling is not matched by a corresponding increased venous drainage. The retrobulbar plexus increases in size, accounting for the forward movement of the globe.

### Clinical management

Treatment of these cases relies not on any regime directed at the eyes but rather therapy of the mass involved. Because these cases are generally associated with an anterior thoracic or cervical mass extensive enough to have enwrapped both jugulars, prognosis can, in this author's opinion at least, be nothing but grave although progression to more severe clinical signs takes a long time.

## Diseases of the cornea

### Corneal ulceration

### Clinical signs

As noted above the rabbit eye is more protuberant than that of many other animals, this giving good vision for almost 360 degrees, essential as a prey species. The problem with this is that the eye is thus more at risk from trauma. Corneal ulceration as a result of trauma from hay or straw in captive environments is thus relatively common

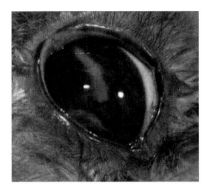

**Figure 4.34**  Linear corneal ulcer from hay awn trauma.

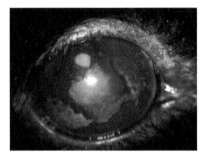

**Figure 4.35**  Non-healing ulcer with ragged non-adherent margin.

(Figure 4.34). In our preliminary study frank corneal ulceration has been seen in 1% of cases examined while chronic superficial stromal scarring, most probably a sequela of previous ulceration, was seen in 1.4% of otherwise normal rabbits. The acute traumatic leisons are normally linear superficial corneal erosions which can best be demarcated with the use of fluorescein as in any species with a corneal abrasive injury. It is important, however, to note the appearance of the ulcer prior to using fluorescein and once fluorescein has been applied to flush it away with sterile water to avoid pooling of dye in an epithelialised corneal facet, in effect a healed ulcer.

Any ulcer requires the three questions: (i) what caused the ulcer? (ii) how deep is it? and (iii) is it healing? As noted previously most post-traumatic rabbit ulcers are superficial, although one caused by an attack from a cage-mate might be deeper and require more aggressive therapy than a superficial ulcer. Even some superficial ulcers may not heal in the few days we should normally expect for a superficial ulcer. Clinical observation in such a case should particularly focus on whether the ulcer margin is clean and crisp, or ragged with superficial stromal oedema underneath the epithelial margin (Figure 4.35). This might suggest the existence of a lip of epithelium, non-adherent to the underlying basement membrane and stroma, impeding healing rather in the same way that the epithelial basement membrane dystrophy prevents healing in so-called boxer ulcers in dogs.

## Aetiopathogenesis

Most superficial ulcers heal within 3–5 days. We probably know more about the rabbit cornea and its healing processes than we do about the dog cornea, since it has been used as an experimental model for many ocular surface conditions. Epithelial cells arise from a stem cell population at the limbus and migrate centrally as basal cells. They then differentiate into wing cells and finally into the squamous cells of the superficial epithelium which are desquamated at a regular rate, probably brushed off the very corneal surface by lid blinks. If the advancing epithelial lip fails to adhere to the underlying basement membrane ulcer healing will be arrested.

Having said that, there is no research on the pathogenesis of these boxer-type non-healing ulcers in the pet rabbit save the clinical anecdote of veterinary ophthalmologists who have treated them, and there is little of that. Is the same pathogenesis underway in the persistent erosion in the rabbit cornea as occurs in the dog [51]? Again here we can point the way to future research. In the meantime, one paper of great value is Stacey Andrew's review in the Veterinary Clinics of America on corneal disease in rabbits [52].

## Clinical management

Debridement of the non-adherent epithelium with a dry cotton bud followed by the use of a tear replacement such as the carbomer-based gel Viscotears may allow epithelial healing to resume. If the underlying basement membrane and stroma are defective, as is the case in Figure 4.36, puncturing this defective tissue by a grid keratotomy can stimulate epithelial healing (Figure 4.37). This technique must be used with caution, however, since the cornea is so much thinner than in the dog, where grid keratotomy is widely practised. Protection of the healing ocular surface is important, either using a bandage contact lens or third eyelid flap for 10 days to 2 weeks after debridment and grid keratotomy.

### Keratitis

Inflammation of the cornea other than that associated with ulceration is not common, but has been noted with an eosinophilic component (Figure 4.38). I hesitate here to divide

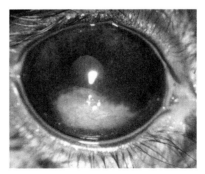

**Figure 4.36** Non-healing ulcer with fibroplastic epithelial defect.

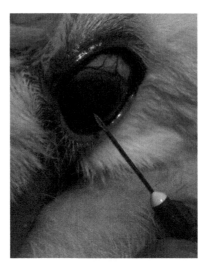

**Figure 4.37**   Grid keratotomy in a non-healing corneal ulcer.

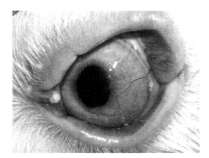

**Figure 4.38**   Eosinophilic keratitis in a rabbit.

the condition into clinical signs, aetiopathogenesis and clinical management; while the proliferative nature of the lesion and the eosinophils seen on taking a surface cytology sample can be illustrated we have no information to give on the aetiology or particularly successful treatment but for an attempt at topical anti-inflammatory treatment with steroid. Keratoconjunctivitis sicca is vanishingly rare in rabbits but diagnosis with a low Schirmer tear test and treatment with tear replacements would be as for other species.

### *Corneal lipidosis*

#### *Clinical signs*

A white opacity in the cornea could be lipid deposition, calcification, inflammatory cell infiltration or scarring. Lipid deposition associated with a systemic increase in circulating through endocrine, genetic [53] or dietary abnormality [54,55] appears as an arc of white at the limbus (Figure 4.39). Crystalline paracentral lipid dystrophy as seen in the dog

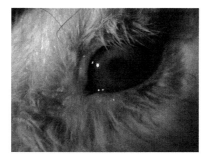

**Figure 4.39**   Arcus lipoides corneae in a rabbit fed milk.

does not appear to have been reported in the rabbit. Other causes of white lesions in the cornea can be corneal oedema seen in glaucoma, of which see more below, or corneal epithelial dystrophy or degeneration [56].

### Aetiopathogenesis

As in any species, the deposition of lipid in the cornea can occur through the death of lipid-laden keratocytes in the central cornea, this giving the signs of an inherited corneal lipid dystrophy. It may, however, occur through the deposition of lipid from the blood, either in the normal cornea, in which case the lipid arcus is seen around the corneal limbus termed arcus lipoides corneae (Figure 4.39), or in association with pathological vasculature, in which case the condition is known as a lipid keratopathy.

## Dermoid

### Clinical signs

As in any species a dysplastic area of cornea with skin elements such as hairs is readily diagnosed as a dermoid. The condition appears to have been reported but once in the veterinary literature [57] but this paucity of evidence may not reflect such a rarity but merely under-reporting.

### Aetiopathogenesis

This sporadic spontaneous congenital defect has no clear aetiological factor in the same way that dermoids in Birman cats appear to be an inherited trait or those in Goldenhaar's syndrome in man are linked to a wider syndrome of defective development.

### Clinical management

The standard treatment for cornea dermoids is removal by superficial keratectomy, but in the case of the rabbit, as with any small exotic species, the thin nature of the cornea renders this an operation best performed by a specialist with access to an operating microscope.

# Diseases of the lens

## *Cataract*

### *Clinical signs*

Cataract is less common in the rabbit than in the guinea pig [58] but can occur in several forms: congenital opacities, most often nuclear in nature with a circular lesion in the centre of the lens, or as a posterior capsular plaque (Figure 4.40). This can be difficult to differentiate from the nuclear opacity but careful observation will allow one to see that it moves in relation to the centre of the lens as the eye rotates or as the observer scans a light beam across the eye. In older animals age-related cataract can be noted but is generally seen in the posterior cortex as small focal dots or lines. On occasion the lens is rapidly opacified to a mature total cataract (Figure 4.41) and while this can be related to diabetes or trauma, there is sometimes no concurrent disease nor a history or other signs of ocular trauma [59].

In our study 17% of rabbits were noted to have some degree of lens opacity ranging from posterior cortical lines through posterior subcapsular plaques through to total

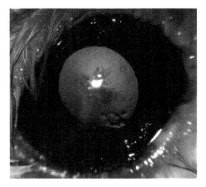

**Figure 4.40**  Posterior capsular plaque cataract in a rabbit.

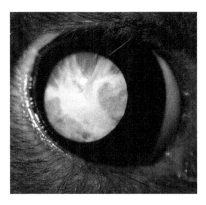

**Figure 4.41**  Mature cataract, rapidly forming, in a rabbit.

mature cataract. Prevalence of cataract increased with age, with 50% of the population having cataract not until 8 years of age.

The more important cataract in rabbits is that associated with *Encephalitozoon cuniculi*, a microsporidial protozoal parasite. In those cases often there is concurrent lens-induced uveitis, often seen as a white mass in the iris but sometimes observed as a vascularised iris lesion, as discussed further under uveitis. This form of cataract and uveitis was seen only in four cases in the thousand animals examined in our study so while the prevalence of *E. cuniculi* seropositivity is relatively high, the involvement of the eye would seem relatively low in the general population.

### Aetiopathogenesis

Any cataract arises as a consequence of disruption of the highly regular arrangement of crystallin proteins in the lens cortex and nucleus or cellular proliferation at the posterior capsule of the lens with underlying subcapsular cortex. This loss of regularity often arises from proteins cross-linking, aggregating and coming out of solution, the very solution that keeps them in regular arranagement preserving transparency. This can happen in age-related cataract because of photo-oxidation of thiol groups of these crystallins to form disulphide bridges between crystallin molecules. Alternatively in congenital cataracts it may be that a genetic mutation in a crystallin molecule leads to loss of solubility of the crystallin protein and its precipitation from solution.

The mechanism by which the protozoan *Encephalitozoon cunilculi* causes cataract is unclear in detail, but its lifecycle gives clues as to the aetiopathogenesis of cataract. The parasite is transmitted between adult rabbits most commonly by ingestion of urine. But passage of parasite between adult and young happens *in utero* with the parasite circulating in the fetus and sometimes ending up residing in the developing lens [60]. At some point in the development of the parasite it migrates through the lens causing opacification. On occasion the parasite migrates through the anterior lens capsule causing liberation of lens protein into the anterior chamber and subsequent development of lens-induced uveitis, covered further below.

### Clinical management

It has to be said that many rabbits with cataracts, even ones blinded by bilateral lens opacification, lead an apparently normal life, able to negotiate around their environment, feed and interact with fellow cage-mates without difficulty. In cases where clinical or financial constraints prevent cataract removal, owners can be reassured that they are unlikely to be compromising their pet's welfare unduly by retaining them blind. Having said that removal of the opacified lens by phacoemulsification is certainly possible, although placement of an intraocular lens in a clinical case has yet to be reported in this species (Figure 4.42).

One problem with removal of the lens by phacoemulsification is that regeneration of lens material is a recognised biological event in rabbit with lenses removed. In dogs the problem of posterior capsular opacification occurs after cataract surgery when the last few remaining cortical lens fibre cells regenerate to give a secondary cataract. In rabbits

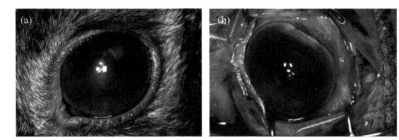

**Figure 4.42**   A rabbit eye with an *Encephalitozoon cuniculi* uveitis and cataract (a) before and (b) after phacoemulsification. Courtesy Dr E. Adkins.

the situation is somewhat different in that the cells of the lens capsule de-differentiate into new lens fibre cells which can then duplicate to can fill the lens capsule with lens material *de novo*. Indeed it was the rabbit in which this phenomenon of lens regeneration was first discovered in mammals, back in 1825. The lens can completely regenerate from the dorsal root of the iris in newts and the lartval cornea in amphibians such as *Xenopus laevis* but the meticulous research of Cocteau and Leroy d'Etoile in the Academy of Surgery in Paris first showed complete lens regeneration from lens capsule in the rabbit [61].

Having said that, lens removal by phacoemulsification is possible and has been suggested as the best treatment for *E. cuniculi*-related opacities [62]. Some would argue that implanting an intraocular lens can prevent posterior capsular opacification while others caution that lens regrowth may force an intraocular lens out of the lens capsular bag with disastrous effects on the otherwise quiet and comfortable eye.

### *Lens luxation*

The majority of lens luxations in the rabbit are secondary to zonular tension in a mature cataract. Primary lens luxation with a zonular degeneration does not appear to have been reported in the rabbit as in the dog [63].

# Diseases of the iris

## Encephalitozoon-*associated lens induced uveitis*

### *Clinical signs*

*E. cuniculi* uveitis normally presents as a white mass in or near the pupil, sometimes with neovascularisation rendering it red or pink (Figures 4.43 and 4.44). Normally there is evidence of cataract also, as might be expected given the aetiopathogenesis of the uveitis as an inflammatory reaction to lens release into the anterior chamber (see below). These eyes are generally hypotonous with a lower than normal intraocular pressure, this manifested as being below the intraocular pressure in the contralateral

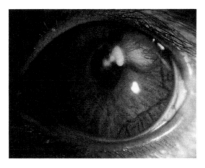

**Figure 4.43**　*E. cuniculi* phacoclastic uveitis with a hyperaemic inflammatory mass and focal anterior capsular cataract.

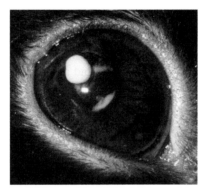

**Figure 4.44**　*E. cuniculi* phacoclastic uveitis with characteristic white inflammatory mass.

eye. In other respects there may be few other signs of uveitis, without miosis, episcleral hyperaemia or other inflammatory changes in the eye such as keratic precipitates or frank hypopyon.

## Aetiopathogenesis

As noted above this protozoal parasite can be transmitted to fetal rabbits *in utero* [64] and be found in the lens, where its migration may cause cataract and later rupture of the anterior lens capsule with liberation of lens material into the anterior chamber. I like to think teleologically of the iris recognising lens material for the first time, given that it has previously been constrained within the lens capsule. It then reacts against this material as a novel antigen and thus produces a uveitis. This may not be strictly true, given that antibodies towards lens antigens can be found in normal individuals as well as those with cataracts [65]. The other unusual feature of this *E. cuniculi*-associated uveitis is that, while it does involve mild hypotony of the eye, other sigs of uveitis such as a miotic pupil, inflammatory cell exudate with keratic precipitates or hypopyon are not generally seen. The lesion classically associated with this specific uveitis in the rabbit, as we noted above, is instead a white circular or ovoid lesion on the surface of the iris.

## Clinical management

It might be argued that, with the pathognomonic appearance of *E. cuniculi*-associated lens-induced uveitis, diagnosis can be by inspection alone. Yet many will want to confirm their suspicions and obtaining a serological titre of circulating antibodies against *E. cuniculi* is sensible before embarking on treatment [66]. A serological titre of 1/32 or greater can be taken as good evidence that *E. cuniculi* infection has occurred but does not prove for certain that the ocular lesions are related to parasitic infection [67]. This is rather an academic splitting of hairs however – the appearance of the lesion in the face of a positive *E. cuniculi* titre should be sufficient for a firm diagnosis. Immunohistochemistry of the affected lens material gives an absolute diagnosis but obviously requires surgery before the sample can be obtained [68].

With regard to clinical management, the original parasiticide used was oral albendazole and this is still a very effective treatment to prevent further progression, athough it does not resolve the lesion. It should be ensured that the albendazole used (normally employed as a sheep wormer) does not have added selenium but only the parasiticide. Fenbendazole, an alternative benzimidazole anthelmintic, is licensed in the UK for use in rabbits with the condition [69]. Topical steroid should be used; a suggested dose is one drop of prednisolone acetate three times daily to control active inflammation while the parasiticide has its effect. Another, more permanent solution, is phacoemulsification to remove the lens and the associated parasites.

## Bacterial iritis

### Clinical signs

The other main cause of intraocular inflammation in rabbits is that caused by a staphylococcal or *Pasteurella* abscessation in the anterior chamber. Intraocular abscessation is generally to be differentiated from *E. cuniculi* uveitis, as described above, by its colour, physical extent and behaviour over time. The *E. cuniculi* uveitic lesion is generally white or pink if vascularisation is pronounced (Figure 4.44). The bacterial iritis is more usually manifest as a yellow mass in the case of *Staphylococcus* (Figure 4.45) or a yellow–white lesion in the case of *Pasteurella*, larger in extent than the *E. cuniculi* lesion, and one

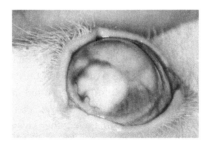

**Figure 4.45**   Staphylococcal panophthalmitis with yellow abscessation.

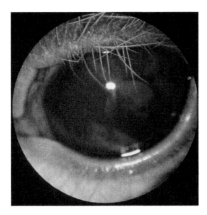

**Figure 4.46**   *Pasteurella* uveitis with miosis, synechiae and hypopyon.

which progresses with time, while the *E. cuniculi* lesion is generally stationary with regards to its extent and progression. *Pasteurella* may give more diffuse iritis with miosis, synechiae, hypopyon and iris swelling and hyperaemia (Figure 4.46) but staphylococcal species more usually give a solitary abscess within the anterior chamber.

### Aetiopathogenesis

Staphylococcal abscesses in rabbits are generally recognised as being haematogenous in origin although local spread can occur. The former method of aetiopathogenesis is probably the case in uveitic staphylococcal involvement. *Pasteurella* may spread haematogeneously or possibly more locally from the nasal mucosa, where it is often considered to be a commensal rather than a pathogen as such, given the number of animals in which it lives in the nasal passages without causing clinical signs.

## Glaucoma

### Clinical signs

As in any other animal species, the diagnosis of glaucoma in the rabbit is primarily based on the finding of increased intraocular pressure by means of tonometry. The use of an applanation tonometer such as the Tonopen is well recognised as valuable in the rabbit but the rebound Tonovet tonometer can also be useful, both because of the much smaller area of contact with the cornea in tonometry and also because local anaesthesia is not needed. Having said that, we do not appear to have a properly calibrated data series for intraocular pressure in the rabbit using either the Tonopen or Tonovet.

Other signs of glaucoma include pupil dilation and episcleral hyperaemia, although in many cases in the rabbit these signs are not as clear-cut as in the dog.

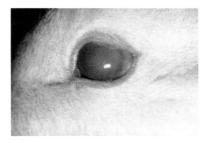

**Figure 4.47**   *bu/bu* inherited buphthalmos in a New Zealand White rabbit.

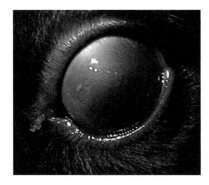

**Figure 4.48**   Glaucoma similar to that in the NZW rabbit but in a pigmented animal.

### Aetiopathogenesis

The most frequently recognised glaucoma in the rabbit population is that associated with the *bu* gene in which early onset gradual enlargement of the globe occurs, often with few other clinical signs (Figure 4.47) [70–72].This gene is noted specifically in the New Zealand White laboratory strain of rabbit but other pet species, presumably with the *bu* gene on board, can manifest the condition in a way identical to that in the white laboratory strain (Figure 4.48). Intraocular pressure rises with blindness ensuing but with little to show that the rabbit is in discomfort or pain [73]. This may, of course, be associated with its behaviour as a prey species where evolution has prevented it from making it obvious that its health is compromised in any way. Yet these animals do not in this author's experience show a reduction in their eating behaviour, nor even the most subtle of signs of depression or lethargy which would in any way signal ocular discomfort such as seen in other species with glaucoma.

The reason for this may be the insidious onset of the disease. As in human patients with POAG, progressive open angle glaucoma, there are no signs of disease until very late in the progression of the condition, unless measurement of visual fields by perimetry is undertaken.

Other causes of increased intraocular pressure include uveitis, in which inflammatory debris can block the iridocorneal angle. While in most cases of uveitis a lower pressure

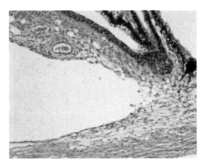

**Figure 4.49**   Histopathology of the normal iridocorneal angle.

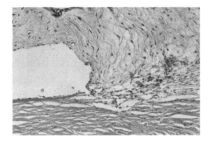

**Figure 4.50**   Histopathology of the angle in a *bu/bu* homozygous rabbit, showing aberrant tissue blocking aqueous drainage.

is noted, this increased intraocular pressure occurs later in life than the *bu*-associated disease and is seen in the context of inflammatory anterior segment disease.

The *bu* gene produces a congenital abnormality of tissue occluding the iridocorneal angle, where aqueous humour normally drains from the eye (Figure 4.49). The normal iridocorneal angle is open with obvious pathways for fluid drainage from the anterior chamber between the cornea and the iris, through the ciliary cleft and out to the episcleral drainage vessels. In *bu*-associated glaucoma a large mass of undifferentiated tissue, which would normally have degenerated *in utero* to open the drainage pathway, remains to block outflow (Figure 4.50). Because this is a congenital defect, intraocular pressure rises early in the young rabbit's life, and with the thin nature of the sclera the eye rapidly increases in size, hence the term buphthalmos and the gene designation *bu*.

As with all glaucoma, while the pressure-raising pathology may be at the iridocorneal angle, the blinding pathology is at the level of the optic nerve head. Intraocular pressure forces the lamina cribrosa, the weakest part of the sclera, outwards, causing disc cupping (Figure 4.51). The ganglion cell axons which course over the edge of this nerve head cup are damaged by the high intraocular pressure slowing axonal transport and causing ganglion cell death through apoptosis.

The *bu* gene is recessive and also has other effects quite apart form its ocular pathology. Homozygous rabbits also show reduced litter size, though the pathological processes that cause intrauterine fetal death are unclear.

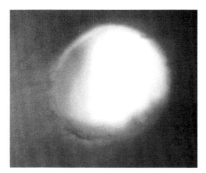

**Figure 4.51**   Optic nerve cupping in rabbit glaucoma.

*Clinical management*

Recognition of the condition takes into account the history of the individual, with regard to species and time of onset of disease. Diagnosis relies on a finding of increased intraocular pressure by tonometry, although even without this increased globe size can lead to the tentative diagnosis. With regard to *bu/bu*-associated glaucoma no treatment to reduce the intraocular pressure at a stage when blindness can be avoided is rarely possible. By time the increased intraocular pressure is noted the animal will have begun the path to increased globe size and resulting blindness [74]. There are ophthalmologists who would suggest long-term medical management of the increased intraocular pressure or placement of a drainage device to provide an artificial pathway for fluid flow out of the eye. In reality, given that there seems little change in behaviour of rabbits with increased intraocular pressure, one might suggest that such heroic therapeutic measures are directed at treating the owner rather than the rabbit – but perhaps that is a little unfair!

# Retinal disease

*Clinical signs*

It might be considered unusual that retinal degenerations equivalent to progressive retinal atrophy in the dog and cat or retinitis pigmentosa in man have only apparently been reported once in the rabbit [75]. Perhaps the lack of a tapetum means that retinal atrophy, so readily detected through tapetal hyper-reflectivity and retinal vessel attenuation in the dog, has not readily been recognised in the rabbit. One inherited retinal degeneration has been reported but without subsequent investigation to determine its phenotypic characteristics or genotypic origins.

# References

1. Bagley LH, Lavach D. Ophthalmic diseases in rabbits. California Vet 1985;49:7–9.
2. Harkness JE, Wagner JE. *The Biology and Medicine of Rabbits and Rodents*, 3rd ed. Philadelphia, PA: Lea and Febiger, 1989.

3. Jeong MB, Kim NR, Yi NY, Park SA, Kim MS, Park JH, Jeong SM, Seo KD, Nam TC, Oh YS, Won MH, Seo KM. Spontaneous ophthalmic diseases in 586 New Zealand white rabbits. Exp Anim 2005;54:395–403.

4. Burling K, Murphy CJ, Curiel JS, Koblick P and Bellhorn RW. Anatomy of the rabbit nasolacrimal duct and its clinical implications. Prog Vet Comp Ophthalmol 1991;1: 33–40.

5. Prince JH. (ed.) *The Rabbit in Eye Research.* Springfield, IL: Charles C Thomas, 1954.

6. Bito LZ. Species differences in the responses of the eye to irritation and trauma: a hypothesis of divergence in ocular defense mechanisms, and the choice of experimental animals for eye research. Exp Eye Res 1984;39:807–829.

7. Ninomiya H, Inomata T, Kanemaki N. Microvascular architecture of the rabbit eye: a scanning electron microscopic study of vascular corrosion casts. J Vet Med Sci 2008;70:887–892.

8. De Schaepdrijver L, Simoens P, Lauwers H, De Geest JP. Retinal vascular patterns in domestic animals. Res Vet Sci 1989;47:34–42.

9. Ruskell GL. Blood vessels of the orbit and globe. In: Prince JH. (ed.) *The Rabbit in Eye Research.* Springfield, IL: Charles C Thomas, 1954, pp. 514–553.

10. Pak MA. Ocular refraction and visual contrast sensitivity of the rabbit, determined by the VECP. Vision Res 1984;24:341–345.

11. de Graauw JG, van Hof MW. Frontal myopia in the rabbit. Behav Brain Res 1980;1: 339–341.

12. de Graauw JG, van Hof MW. Relation between behavior and eye-refraction in the rabbit. Physiol Behav 1978;21(2):257–259.

13. Van Hof MW. Visual acuity in the rabbit. Vision Res 1967;7:749–751.

14. Vaney DI. The grating acuity of the wild European rabbit. Vision Res 1980;20:87–89.

15. van Wyk M, Taylor WR, Vaney DI. Local edge detectors: a substrate for fine spatial vision at low temporal frequencies in rabbit retina. J Neurosci 2006;26:13250–13263.

16. Davis FA. The anatomy and histology of the eye and orbit of the rabbit. Trans Am Ophthal Soc 1929;27:401–441.

17. Nuboer JFW. Spectral discrimination in a rabbit. Doc Ophthalmol 1971;30:279–298.

18. Juliusson B, Bergström A, Röhlich P, Ehinger B, van Veen T, Szél A. Complementary cone fields of the rabbit retina. Invest Ophthalmol Vis Sci 1994;35:811–818.

19. Jones SM, Carrington SD. Pasteurella dacryocystitis in rabbits. Vet Rec 1988;122:514–515.

20. Florin M, Rusanen E, Haessig M, Richter M, Spiess BM. Clinical presentation, treatment, and outcome of dacryocystitis in rabbits: a retrospective study of 28 cases (2003–2007). Vet Ophthalmol 2009;12:350–356.

21. Anon. Nasolacrimal duct lavage in rabbits. Lab Anim (NY) 2006;35:22–24.

22. Marini RP, Foltz CJ, Kersten D, Batchelder M, Kaser W, Li X. Microbiologic, radiographic, and anatomic study of the nasolacrimal duct apparatus in the rabbit (*Oryctolagus cuniculus*). Lab Anim Sci 1996;46:656–662.

23. Barandun G, Palmer D. Epiphora in dwarf rabbits. Anatomic, clinical and pathologicoanatomic studies of the lacrimal canal in the dwarf rabbit. Tierarztl Prax 1980;10:403–410.

24. Harcourt-Brown F. Calcium deficiency, diet and dental disease in pet rabbits. Vet Rec 1996;139:567–571.

25. Harcourt-Brown FH. Dental disease in pet rabbits 1. Normal dentition, pathogenesis and aetiology. In Practice 2009;31:370–379.

26. Harcourt-Brown FH. Dental disease in pet rabbits 2. Diagnosis and treatment. In Practice 2009;31:432–445.

27. Cooper SC, McLellan GJ, Rycroft AN. Conjunctival flora observed in 70 healthy domestic rabbits (*Oryctolagus cuniculus*). Vet Rec 2001;149:232–235.

28. Snyder SB, Fox JG, Campell LH, Soave OA. Disseminated staphylococcal disease in laboratory rabbits (*Oryctolagus cuniculus*). Lab Anim Sci 1976;26:86–88.

29. Abrams KL, Brooks DE, Funk RS, Theran P. Evaluation of the Schirmer tear test in clinically normal rabbits. Am J Vet Res 1990;51:1912–1913

30. Shirani D, Selk Ghaffari M, Akbarein H, Haji Ali Asgari A. Effects of short-term oral administration of trimethoprim-sulfamethoxazole on Schirmer II tear test results in clinically normal rabbits. Vet Rec 2010;166:623–624.

31. Srivastava KK, Pick JR, Johnson PT. Characterisation of a *Hemophilus* sp. isolated from a rabbit with conjunctivitis. Lab Anim 1986;36:291–293.

32. Hinton M. Treatment of purulent staphylococcal conjunctivitis in rabbits with autogenous vaccine. Lab Anim 1977;11:163–164.

33. Matros LE, Ansari MM, Van Pelt CS. Eye anomaly in a dwarf rabbit. Avian Exotic Pract 1986;3:13–14.

34. Bauck L. Ophthalmic conditions in pet rabbits and rodents. Comp Cont Educ Pract Vet 1989;11:258–268.

35. Dupont, C, Carrier M, Gauvin J. Bilateral precorneal membranous occlusion in a dwarf rabbit. J Small Exotic Anim Med 1995;3:41–44.

36. Roze M, Ridings B, Lagadic M. Comparative morphology of epicorneal conjunctival membranes in rabbits and human pterygium. Vet Ophthalmol 2001;4:171–174.

37. Donnelly TM, Fisher PG, Lackner PA. Epicorneal membrane on the eye of a Rex rabbit. Lab Anim 2002;31:23–25.

38. Allgoewer I, Malho P, Schulze H, Schäffer E. Aberrant conjunctival stricture and overgrowth in the rabbit. Vet Ophthalmol 2008;11:18–22.

39. Millichamp NJ, Collins BR. Blepharoconjunctivitis associated with *Staphylococcus aureus* in a rabbit. J Am Vet Med Assoc 1986;189:1153–1154.

40. Zúñiga MC. A pox on thee! Manipulation of the host immune system by myxoma virus and implications for viral-host co-adaptation.Virus Res 2002;88:17–33.

41. Janssens G, Simoens P, Muylle S, Lauwers H. Bilateral prolapse of the deep gland of the third eyelid in a rabbit: diagnosis and treatment. Lab Anim Sci 1999;49:105–109.

42. Roxburgh G, Boydell P, Genovese L. Prolapse and hyperplasia of a third eyelid gland in 4 rabbits. J Br Assoc Vet Ophthalmol 1998;12:4.

43. Morgan RV, Duddy JM, McClurg K. Prolapse of the gland of the third eyelid in dogs: a retrospective study of 89 cases (1980 to 1990). J Am Anim Hosp Assoc 1993;29:56–60.

44. Stanley RG, Kaswan RL. Modification of the orbital rim anchorage method for surgical replacement of the gland of the third eyelid in dogs. J Am Vet Med Assoc 1994;205:1412–1414.

45. Nielsen JN, Carlton WW. Colobomatous microphthalmos in a New Zealand white rabbit, arising from a colony with suspected vitamin E deficiency. Lab Anim Sci 1995;45:320–322.

46. O'Reilly A, McCowan C, Hardman C, Stanley R. Taenia serialis causing exophthalmos in a pet rabbit. Vet Ophthalmol 2002;5:227–230.

47. Volopich S, Gruber A, Hassan J, Hittmair KM, Schwendenwein I, Nell B. Malignant B-cell lymphoma of the Harder's gland in a rabbit. Vet Ophthalmol 2005;8:259–263.

48. Oryan A, Zaker SR. Effects of topical application of honey on cutaneous wound healing in rabbits. Zentralbl Veterinarmed A 1998;45:181–188.

49. Wagner F, Beinecke A, Fehr M, Brunkhorst N, Mischke R, Gruber AD. Recurrent bilateral exophthalmos associated with metastatic thymic carcinoma in a pet rabbit. J Small Anim Pract 2005;46:393–397.

50. Vernau KM, Grahn BH, Clarke-Scott HA, Sullivan N. Thymoma in a geriatric rabbit with hypercalcemia and periodic exophthalmos. J Am Vet Med Assoc 1995;206:820–822.

51. Gelatt KN, Samuelson DA. Recurrent corneal erosions in the boxer dog. J Am Anim Hosp Assoc 1982;18:453–460.

52. Andrew SE. Corneal diseases of rabbits. Vet Clin North Am Exot Anim Pract 2002;5:341–356.

53. Garibaldi BA, Goad ME. Lipid keratopathy in the Watanabe (WHHL) rabbit. Vet Pathol 1988; 25:173–174.

54. Sebesteny A, Sheraidah GA, Trevan DJ, Alexander RA, Ahmed AI. Lipid keratopathy and atheromatosis in an SPF laboratory rabbit colony attributable to diet. Lab Anim 1985;19: 180–188.

55. Gwin RM, Gelatt KN. Bilateral ocular lipidosis in a cottontail rabbit fed an all-milk diet. J Am Vet Med Assoc 1977;171:887–889.

56. Port CD, Dodd DC. Two cases of corneal epithelial dystrophy in rabbits. Lab Anim Sci 1983;33:587–588.

57. Wagner F, Brügmann M, Drommer W, Fehr M. Corneal dermoid in a dwarf rabbit (*Oryctolagus cuniculi*). Contemp Top Lab Anim Sci 2000;39:39–40.

58. Williams DL, Sullivan A. Ocular disease in the guinea pig (*Cavia porcellus*): a survey of 1000 animals. Vet Ophthalmol 2010;13:54–62.

59. Munger RJ, Langevin N, Podval J. Spontaneous cataracts in laboratory rabbits. Vet Ophthalmol 2002;5:177–181.

60. Ashton N, Cook C, Clegg F. Encephalitozoonosis (nosematosis) causing bilateral cataract in a rabbit. Br J Ophthalmol 1976;60:618–631.

61. Gwon A. Lens regeneration in mammals: a review. Survey Ophthalmol 2006;51:51–62.

62. Felchle LM, Sigler RL. Phacoemulsification for the management of *Encephalitozoon cuniculi*-induced phacoclastic uveitis in a rabbit. Vet Ophthalmol 2002;5:211–215.

63. Curtis R, Barnett KC, Lewis SJ. Clinical and pathological observations concerning the aetiology of primary lens luxation in the dog. Vet Rec 1983;112:238–246.

64. Baneux PJ, Pognan F. In utero transmission of *Encephalitozoon cuniculi* strain type I in rabbits. Lab Anim 2003;37:132–138.

65. van der Woerdt A, Nasisse MP, Davidson MG. Lens-induced uveitis in dogs: 151 cases (1985–1990). J Am Vet Med Assoc 1992;201:921–926.

66. Thalhammer JG, Joachim A. Clinical symptoms and diagnosis of encephalitozoonosis in pet rabbits. Vet Parasitol 2008;151:115–124.

67. Harcourt-Brown FM, Holloway HK. Encephalitozoon cuniculi in pet rabbits. Vet Rec 2003;152:427–431.

68. Giordano C, Weigt A, Vercelli A, Rondena M, Grilli G, Giudice C. Immunohistochemical identification of *Encephalitozoon cuniculi* in phacoclastic uveitis in four rabbits. Vet Ophthalmol 2005;8:271–275.

69. Suter C, Müller-Doblies UU, Hatt JM, Deplazes P. Prevention and treatment of *Encephalitozoon cuniculi* infection in rabbits with fenbendazole. Vet Rec 2001;148:478–480.

70. Hanna BL, Sawin PB, Sheppars LB. Buphthalmia in the rabbit. J Heredity 1962; 62:294–299.

71. Tesluk G, Peiffer RL, Brown D. A clinical and pathological study of inherited glaucoma in New Zealand white rabbits. Lab Anim 1982;16:234–239.

72. Künzel F, Gruber A, Tichy A, Edelhofer R, Nell B, Hassan J, Leschnik M, Lee PF. Gonioscopic study of hereditary buphthalmia in rabbits. Arch Ophthalmol 1968;79:775–778.

73. Kolker AE, Moses RA, Constant MA, Becker B. The development of glaucoma in rabbits. Invest Ophthalmol 1963;2:316–321.

74. Vareilles P, Coquet P, Lotti VJ. Intraocular pressure responses to antiglaucoma agents in spontaneous buphthalmic rabbits. Ophthalmol Res 1980;12:2296–2302.

75. Reichenbach A, Baar U. Retinitis-pigmentosa-like tapetoretinal degeneration in a rabbit breed. Doc Ophthalmol 1985;60:71–78.

# Chapter 5

# The guinea pig eye

## Anatomy and physiology of the guinea pig eye

The guinea pig eye is not dissimilar to that of other rodents of similar size but with one major difference, that of the retinal vasculature which is paurangiotic but to a degree where, by fundoscopy, the retina appears devoid of blood vessels. This has implications for oxygenation of the retina but not for the acuity of guinea pig vision, as we see below. The retina may thus, with its lack of blood vessels, appear to the uninitiated as if it were suffering from an atrophic degeneration. But other than that the eye appears unremarkable. What is, however, quite remarkable and with potential effects on the lens and retina, is that the guinea pig is incapable of synthesising its own vitamin C. The vast majority of cavy owners are well aware of this fact and supplement their pet's diet. Having said that, our recent study of 1000 guinea pigs shows that 45% had some ocular anomaly, many of them lens-related [1]. Our study of eyes of 1000 rabbits (see Chapter 5) shows a very much lower prevalence of eye and lens abnormalities, so it is possible that, even when supplemented, these guinea pigs are subject to levels of dietary ascorbate sufficiently low to lead to lens opacities. Such a wild assertion clearly needs further investigation, but the high levels of ocular abnormalities in otherwise normal healthy guinea pigs is surprising.

## What do guinea pigs see?

Guinea pigs are a highly visual species, using sight from the moment of their precocious birth and reaching a visual acuity of 2.7 cycles per degree (cpd), the equivalent of a Snellen acuity of around 6/70, although it has to be said that this figure was obtained by histological determination of photoreceptor density and not from retinoscopy or behavioural testing of acuity [2,3]. There are of course other factors involved in visual acuity other than the retinal photoreceptor and ganglion cell density. A key one is the refractive state of the eye and here interesting recent research has shown that a normal group of 220 guinea pigs demonstrated an average hypermetropic (long-sighted) refraction at 3 weeks of age of +2.3 D but with a wide variation and a standard deviation of 4.1 D; a number of animals were significantly myopic (short-sighted) [4]. This was wider than the variation in a previous study but with a similar mean of 4.8 D. Twenty-eight of the 220 animals in Jiang's study [3] were selected as being bilaterally myopic or anisometropic where one eye is short-sighted and the other either emetropic – normally sighted – or myopic. These animals were found to be spontaneously myopic at between -15.7 D and -1.5 D even though the animals were visual as determined by optomotor studies. Albino guinea pigs have been shown to develop a high degree of myopia [6]. Howlett and McFadden's [5] guinea pigs, however, did not develop this high myopia so it remains unclear exactly how well guinea pigs kept as pets do see, especially given the high prevalence of ocular defects, as we will see below.

## Diseases of the guinea pig eye

### *Microphthalmos and anophthalmos*

#### *Clinical signs*

As with any species, sporadic congenital abnormalities in globe size are seen in the guinea pig on occasion. Given that neonatal guinea pigs are precocious and born with their eyes open, abnormally small eyes are obvious from birth, especially as they may be associated with mucopurulent discharge which builds up as the orbit is, relatively speaking, overly large for the globe situated within it. Entropion can occur in such cases as the ocular surface is recessed given the small size of the eye. Guinea pigs can be born with no apparent globe whatsoever (Figure 5.1). These may be termed anophthalmic, although many will have a small ocular remnant and so should properly be termed extreme microphthalmic.

#### *Aetiopathogenesis*

The association between the lens and the development of the globe means that animals with congenital cataracts may well also be affected by microphthalmos. This is particu-

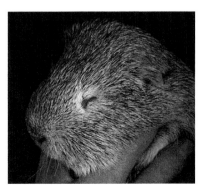

**Figure 5.1**   Guinea pig with congenital anophthalmos.

larly true in Roan x Roan crosses. Experimental studies have shown anophthalmos in offspring of rodents treated with the fungicide benomyl and, while this is unlikely to be the cause of globe abnormalities in pet animals, this is just one example of a chemical causing this deformity. Nutritional causes include hypovitamosis A, as seen in piglets although not reported in guinea pigs. Similarly we know of inherited defects in globe size in other species and so microphthalmos or anophthalmos may have a genetic predisposition [7].

### Clinical management

Clearly microphthalmos and anophthalmos cannot be cured, but clinical management should include an evaluation of possible causes, as noted above. Management of the condition may include topical antibiotic to control possible infection in the unoccupied orbit in these animals. In a severely microphthalmic animal entropion and subsequent irritation caused by trichiasis with hair abrading the ocular surface may need to be managed by Hotz–Celsus surgery, although dealing with in-turning caused by lack of a suitably sized globe can be taxing.

## Entropion

### Clinical signs

Entropion (Figure 5.2) is seen when the hairless lid margin is not appreciated since the lid in-turning leads haired skin to be apposed against the corneal surface. Blepharospasm and excess lacrimation are seen and ocular surface pain may be sufficient on occasion to cause inappetance and lethargy.

### Aetiopathogenesis

Lid in-turning may be associated with an abnormally small globe, as noted above, or with a defect in the tarsal plate of the lid as seen in several dog breeds. It may occur secondary to the irritation caused by conjunctivitis, keratoconjunctivitis sicca or trichi-

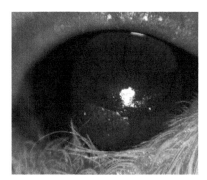

**Figure 5.2**  Guinea pig with entropion.

asis; these are covered further below. The condition becomes a problem when in-turning is sufficient to cause the lid hair to abrade on the corneal surface, often with resultant corneal ulceration.

### Clinical management

It is important to determine the cause of the lid in-turning and to address this before attempting to correct the lid in-turning. This can be achieved through a standard Hotz–Celsus surgery where a strip of eyelid skin is removed and the resulting defect sutured closed. The guinea pig has a thin delicate lid and only 1 mm or so need be removed to correct the lid in-turning, thus this surgery requires magnification with a head loupe at least and fine ophthalmic surgical equipment.

## Trichiasis

### Clinical signs

Rex and Texel breeds with their bristly coats are predisposed to ocular surface abrasion in the first few hours of life (Figure 5.3). Irritation caused by this abrasion and often the resulting corneal ulceration, goes on to cause further blepharospasm and lid in-turning, with further ocular surface abrasion. In other more smooth-haired breeds trichiasis can occur with entropion, with the ocular surface abrasion again leading to a worsening of the irritation.

### Aetiopathogenesis

The Texel breed has been created specifically with this bristly coated appearance and, in this breed, as with pedigree dogs, specific breeding for unusual conformation may compromise welfare.

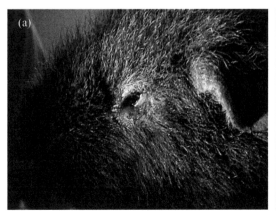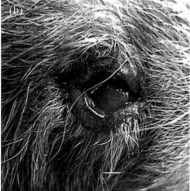

**Figure 5.3**    (a, b) Texel guinea pig with trichiasis.

### Clinical management

Texel and to some extent Rex breeders know the importance of ensuring that the periocular hair in neonates does not abrade the ocular surface. They use petrolatum jelly to ensure that the short hairs at the eyelid margin do not cause lesions on the corneal surface. In cases where this care at birth has not been taken, it can be very difficult to manage the resulting corneal pathology. Lubricating the eye with a tear replacement gel may relieve discomfort as may a topical non-steroidal agent such as ketorolac (Acular; Allergan). Long-term corneal ulceration and oedema may be unavoidable in severe cases.

## Dermoid

### Clinical signs

One of the joys of comparative ophthalmology is that many conditions are essentially similar across species. A dermoid, the aberrant development of a dermal area, often haired, on the otherwise transparent cornea, is exactly such a condition. Whether in the dog, the cow or the guinea pig, a dermoid is essentially identical. Most are haired lesions on the cornea although aberrant adnexal haired tissue growths may occur alone or with a corneal lesion (Figure 5.4).

### Aetiopathogenesis

There is evidence of inheritance of a propensity to develop dermoids; German shepherd dogs are more likely to develop the condition and dermoids are seen in the recessive Goldenhaar's syndrome in man. Whether this is true in guinea pigs is unclear.

### Clinical management

Simple removal of these lesions by superficial keratectomy is curative. The difficulty in guinea pigs is the very nature of the cornea. While in the dog or horse superficial

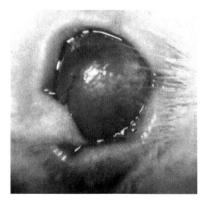

**Figure 5.4**   Guinea pig with dermoid.

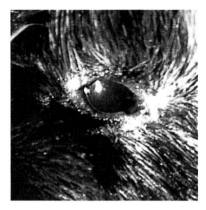

**Figure 5.5**   Conjunctivitis in a guinea pig.

keratectomy is not difficult because of the thickness of the cornea, in the guinea pig the cornea no thicker than 500 µm so there is little tissue to remove. Thankfully the dermal tissue of the dermoid can normally be removed from the underlying cornea, although magnification and microsurgical equipment such as a Colibri forceps and Castroveijo corneal scissors are essential.

## Conjunctivitis

### Clinical signs

Conjunctival irritation and inflammation may vary from a mild hyperaemia, through conujnctival hyperplasia (Figure 5.5) or chemosis (although this seems to be relatively rare in guinea pigs), to frank purulent discharge. It is important to differentiate this from the white cell-free fluid which is naturally produced by the guinea pig eye and aids with grooming (see below). Blepharospasm may occur concurrently. Conjunctivitis may occur with keratitis or alone, depending on the causative agent.

### Aetiopathogenesis

Chlamydial conjunctivitis is widely reported in the literature but this is probably because it is a model for human chlamydial keratoconjunctivitis rather than it necessarily being a common cause in companion animal disease. Guinea pigs can also develop a severe keratoconjunctivitis associated with *Listeria monocytogenes*. Other Gram-negative bacteria such as *Salmonella* have been reported as causative agents in guinea pig conjunctivitis. Sterile conjunctivitis may also be seen where poor quality hay is used with an unacceptably high dust level. Indeed the most common cause of conjunctivitis is probably a foreign body such as a hay awn (Figure 5.5). Conjunctival inflammation is one of the earliest signs of vitamin C deficiency, a potentially severe condition in this species.

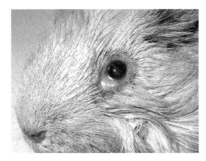

**Figure 5.6**   White fluid secretion is a normal finding in some guinea pig eyes.

## Clinical management

Evaluation of a cases of conjunctivitis in the guinea pig should aim to determine the cause, assessing the possibility that environmental agents such as a hay awn foreign body, dust from poor quality hay, or dietary factors such as a low level of vitamin C are instrumental in causing the condition. Where no obvious physical cause can be elucidated, an infectious agent maybe implicated. While bacteriological investigation may be considered worthwhile, financial constraints will preclude such evaluation in many cases, and use of a broad-spectrum topical antibiotic will, if successful, provide a diagnostic and therapeutic step in one. In cases where such an immediate course of action does not succeed, it may be well worth taking samples for bacteriology but in such cases culture or polymerase chain reaction (PCR) for *Chlamydia* should also be included.

Where *Chlamydia* is isolated or suspected, topical tetracycline ointment should be employed and, if this is successful in ameliorating conjunctival signs, doxycycline might be considered to ensure that the infectious agent does not continue to reside in the nasopharynx.

Dacryocystitis does not seem to occur in the guinea pig with anything like the frequency it does in the rabbit, but unresponsive purulent discharge should always alert one to the fact that this may be the underlying lesion. As noted above guinea pigs can normally produce a milky white ocular secretion (Figure 5.6) which is said to lubricate the eye and aid in cleaning the face. To date we have little or no information on the composition of this fluid nor on its origin or function.

## Keratoconjuctivitis sicca

### Clinical signs

Signs of ocular irritation and, in particular partial closure of the palpebral aperture, together with a lack of clear sharp reflection of light form the ocular surface are highly suggestive of clinical dry eye (Figure 5.7). A Schirmer tear test is the standard method of evaluating tear production (Figure 5.8). The normal Schirmer tear test has been reported as a median of 3 mm/min with a range of 0–12 mm/min in one study of 31 healthy guinea pigs of various ages and breeds [8]. An earlier study on 28 2.5-year-old

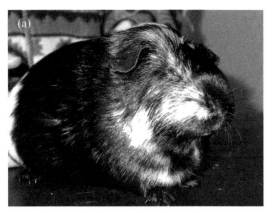
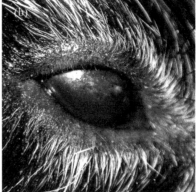

**Figure 5.7**  (a, b) Keratoconjunctivitis sicca in a guinea pig. Note the lustreless ocular surface.

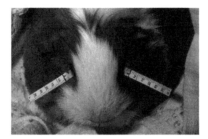

**Figure 5.8**  Schirmer tear test in a guinea pig with unilateral dry eye.

Dunkin-Hartley guinea pigs reported a mean Schirmer tear test before topical anaesthesia of $0.36 \pm 1.1$ mm/min and $0.43 \pm 1.29$ mm/min after topical anaesthesia but these exceptionally low measurements of tear production may be a function of choosing one breed of cavy at one age [9]. Corneal touch threshold as measured with a Cochon et Bonnet anaesthesiometer in that study was between 3.7 and 6.4 g/mm$^2$ in different areas of the cornea, again significantly different from that measured by the study of a wider range of guinea pig breeds where the mean was 6.6 g/mm$^2$ with a range of touch threshold between 3.2 and 17.7 g/mm$^2$. Given the small size of the eye the phenol red thread test may be appropriate, with results of $16 \pm 4.7$ mm wetting in 15 seconds for the Dunkin-Hartley guinea pigs and $21 \pm 4.2$ mm wetting in 15 seconds for the wider range of cavies.

## Aetiopathogenesis

It is unclear whether the same immune-mediated lacrimal destruction occurs in guinea pigs as is the case in the dog but given that topical cyclosporine has a beneficial effect (see below) we might anticipate that the same pathological processes are reducing tear production in these animals as in canine patients.

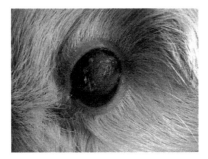

**Figure 5.9**   Traumatic corneal lesion from hay awn.

### Clinical management

We have shown topical cyclosporine (Optimmune, Schering-Plough) to have a beneficial effect in increasing tear production in guinea pigs with dry eye but, given the high price of this medication, it may well be that tear replacement therapy with a carbomer-based gel such as Viscotears (Allergan) or a more liquid medication such as hydroxymethyl-cellulose is a more practical approach.

### Keratitis

### Clinical signs

A common condition in guinea pigs is ocular surface trauma, normally from a hay shard or grass awn (Figure 5.9). In the acute phase a corneal epithelial erosion and sometimes also stromal damage occurs, but with little blepharospasm in the majority of cases. Later changes yield a scar with inflammatory cell infiltrate and fibrosis which often impairs vision but again rarely leads to obvious signs of ocular surface discomfort.

### Aetiopathogenesis

The fact that guinea pigs burrow in straw and leaf litter both in the wild and in captivity renders them prone to such injuries. The lack of obvious reaction to such a nociceptive stimulus means that often such corneal injuries in captive guinea pigs are not noticed by owners until a later stage when the inflammation and fibroplasia are ongoing.

### Clinical management

In the acute phase, removal of the inciting foreign body and provision of topical antibiotic drops or gel, with a broad-spectrum drug such as chloramphenicol or gentamicin, is appropriate. In the chronic phase a superficial keratectomy might be appropriate to remove the reactive tissue from the corneal surface, but this is rarely implemented, especially given the potentially hazardous general anaesthetic required for such surgery.

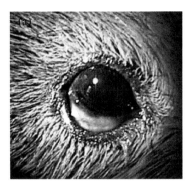
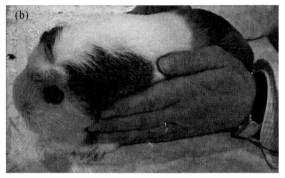

**Figure 5.10** (a) Subconjunctival lipid deposition (fatty eye). (b) Guinea pig 'fattened up' for showing.

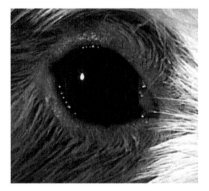

**Figure 5.11** 'Flesh eye' in a guinea pig.

### 'Fatty eye' and 'flesh eye'

#### Clinical signs

These two conditions, with their nomenclature taken straight from guinea pig breeders and showers, involve masses around the eye. Fatty eye is, as its name suggests, a deposition of lipid in the bulbar conjunctiva, appearing as a white or pink–white lesion (Figure 5.10a). Flesh eye, again well named, is probably the equivalent of nictitans gland prolapse in the dog, although to date we have no histological evidence to confirm this. It appears as a pink, or red–pink mass in the medial canthus, quite different from fatty eye (Figure 5.11).

#### Aetiopathogenesis

We have little evidence on the aetiology or even the histological nature of these lesions, but fatty eye is seen in guinea pigs 'fattened up' not for the pot, as they might be in their homeland of Peru, but for shows! Figure 5.10b shows just such an animal. Understandably, having been fed to present a rounded figure, conjunctival lipid deposition is seen relatively commonly.

### Clinical management

Fatty eye can be managed by reducing the calorific dietary input of the animal but reduction in size of the lesion will take time. To date no report exists of removal of the medial canthal mass in flesh eye but we might suppose that removal by sharp dissection might be appropriate.

## Corneal lipidosis

### Clinical signs

Another manifestation of lipid deposition in the eye is corneal lipidosis. This manifests as a circular or oval white area in the central or paracentral cornea (Figure 5.12). At higher magnification it can be seen that the lesion consists of a number of focal white deposits, either granular in appearance or more commonly spicular (Figure 5.13). Each of these is a triglyceride or cholesterol crystal, the former more likely to be small and granular while the cholesterol crystals are somewhat larger and appear as straight spicules.

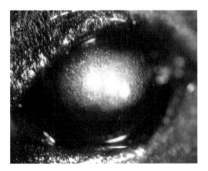

**Figure 5.12**   Dense corneal lipidosis in a guinea pig eye.

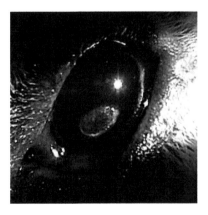

**Figure 5.13**   An ellipse of lipid deposition in a guinea pig eye.

### Aetiopathogenesis

It is unclear to what degree dietary fat plays a role in the genesis of these lesions. Stromal lipid dystrophy in the dog and in man is bilateral and is not associated with an increase in circulating lipid levels, just as is seen in these guinea pigs. Although we have no evidence of the gene involved, it is reasonable, therefore, to consider these lesions to be true stromal lipid dystrophy.

### Clinical management

While we have just said that these lesions are likely to be genetic and not related to excess dietary fat intake, an assiduous veterinarian might reasonably make detailed enquiries with regard to the animal's diet and perhaps also take a fasted blood sample for circulating lipid analysis. Having said this, such lesions, even though they are in the central visual axis of the animal and so should compromise vision quite substantially, seem to make little difference to the animal's quality of life and thus owners should be advised that unless investigations show excess dietary fat intake to be at the root of the problem, there is little that needs to be done to limit the problem, and little to be concerned about.

## Heterotopic bone formation

### Clinical signs

This fascinating condition has a very distinctive appearance, that of a white lesion at the limbus, protruding slightly into the cornea (Figures 5.14 and 5.15). In another species group it might be confused with a lipid deposition but in guinea pigs this well demarcated white deposit is one thing and one thing only – heterotopic bone formation. Some reports have suggested that glaucoma may be seen concurrent with this condition, but this author's experience is that, if anything, intraocular pressure is lower than normal in most of these eyes; little clinical significance can be placed on such a finding, since the eyes generally have no signs of other disease such as uveitis associated with the white

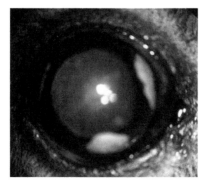

**Figure 5.14**   Small area of heterotopic bone formation.

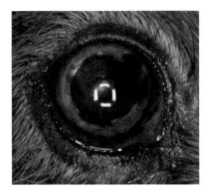

**Figure 5.15**   Extensive limbal heterotopic bone formation.

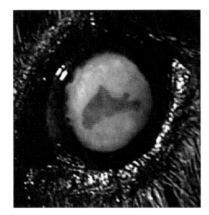

**Figure 5.16**   Heterotopic bone formation of entire globe.

calcium deposit. The point at which the intraocular pressure may rise is in animals where the entire globe is overtaken by this mineral deposition (Figure 5.16), but even here intraocular pressure as measured by tonometry, paradoxically does not seem to rise in most cases.

### Aetiopathogenesis

This condition used to be termed an osseous choristoma [10]. That condition, however, is a benign slow-growing congenital tumour [11] and thus the term is inappropriate for this condition in the guinea pig eye which, while slowly developing, is neither congenital nor a neoplasm. It is, as Brooks reported, heterotopic bone formation in the ciliary body [12]. Others have confirmed Brooks' diagnosis while retaining the term osseous choristoma [13]. The pathogenesis here appears quite remarkable. Ascorbic acid, vitamin C, promotes calcium deposition when at high concentrations in tissue. The ciliary body secretes vitamin C into the aqueous humour, potentially to ensure sufficiently high levels in the lens to prevent cataract formation. High levels at this anatomical location in the eye cause the build-up of calcium at the limbus, causing this heterotopic bone formation. It is unusual, having said this, that the white calcium plaque is generally a focal lesion rather than one which encircles the eye at the level of the limbus although this can occur (Figure 5.15). Why calcium deposition and new bone formation should occur in this focal manner is unclear. There are obviously further lessons to be learned regarding the development of this condition.

### Clinical management

Most cases of heterotopic bone formation do not require treatment, since the appearance of this white plaque, while disconcerting to owners, does not impede vision in the guinea pig or cause any discomfort. The report that glaucoma may supervene might suggest that measurement of intraocular pressure should be central to the management of this condition but in this author's clinical experience glaucoma is unlikely to occur unless the whole globe is overtaken by bone deposition. Given that applanation or rebound tonometry is currently not a technique regularly used in many veterinary practices, unless signs of ocular discomfort, blindness or globe enlargement supervene, an increase in intraocular pressure should not be a prime concern.

## Cataract

### Clinical signs

Lens opacification can range from a small lesion in the nucleus or posterior subcapsular cortex to an obvious complete mature cataract (Figures 5.17–5.19). The opacity may have no effect on vision and only be picked up on a routine ophthalmic examination of an otherwise normal eye, or may be sight threatening or frankly blinding and clear to all who observe the animal. In our study of 1000 animals 40% had some degree of lens

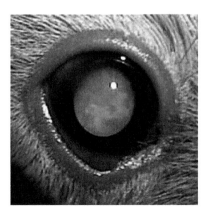

**Figure 5.17**  Mature cataract in diabetic guinea pig also with fatty eye.

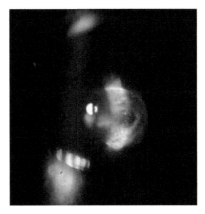

**Figure 5.18**  Posterior polar congenital inherited cataract in one of an entire litter affected.

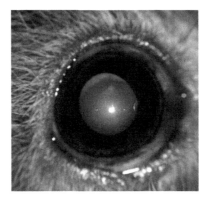

**Figure 5.19**  Nuclear sclerosis with central nuclear cataract in an ageing guinea pig.

opacification, although in the vast majority of these animals no effect on visual acuity was noted [1].

*Aetiopathogenesis*

The fact that guinea pigs require a dietary input of ascorbic acid, and the importance of this vitamin in preventing the oxidative changes at the heart of many cataracts suggests that low levels of vitamin C may be central to the high levels of lens changes we noted in guinea pigs [14]. Having said that no correlation between prevalence of cataract and level of vitamin C supplementation (or lack of it) was noted in our study. It is known that congenital cataract is seen in N13 laboratory guinea pigs as an inherited cataract associated with a crystallin gene mutation, namely a splice-site muta-tion in the zeta crystallin [15]. We have seen a number of other congenital lens opacities in related animals, which are probably associated with other lens protein gene mutations. Diabetic cataract occurs frequently in guinea pigs and presents as a mature lens opacity.

### Clinical management

Any cataract in any species can be removed either by phacoemulsification surgery if the globe is large enough or by irrigation/aspiration if the corneal diameter is too small to accommodate the phaco probe. Thus guinea pig cataracts could be removed but one has to ask whether this is appropriate for the guinea pig as a companion animal pet. What reduction is there in the quality of life of a blind as opposed to a sighted guinea pig? Anecdotal reports of the behaviour of blind guinea pigs compared with sighted ones suggest that there is not a huge difference between the two. Perhaps the potential downside of ocular inflammation and the difficulty of guinea pig anaesthesia for a prolonged surgery such as cataract removal, suggests that the upside of restored vision is not sufficient to justify cataract removal. This is not the sort of comment normally expected of an ophthalmologist but we must be informed by evidence from the behaviour of sighted and blind cavies.

## Retinal anomalies

### Clinical signs

The guinea pig has an anangiotic fundus, one in which there are no retinal blood vessels (Figure 5.20). In addition the guinea pig fundus has no tapetum. These differences from the retina seen in the dog and cat may explain why we have no records of retinal degeneration in the guinea pig. In the dog and cat we see tapetal hyper-reflectivity and reduction in calibre of retinal vessels as key ophthalmic signs of retinal degeneration. But without tapetum or retinal vessels, the key signs of retinal degeneration cannot be seen. Only one report exists of retinal degeneration in the guinea pig but this reduction in retinal function was determined by electroretinography and not fundoscopy or behavioural changes [16].

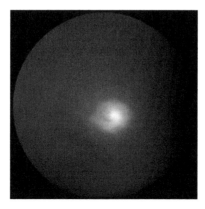

**Figure 5.20**   The anangiotic guinea pig fundus.

# References

1. Williams DL, Sullivan A. Ocular disease in the guinea pig (*Cavia porcellus*): a survey of 1000 animals. Vet Ophthalmol 2010;13:54–62.
2. Buttery RG, Hinrichsen CF, Weller WL, Haight JR. How thick should a retina be? A comparative study of mammalian species with and without intraretinal vasculature. Vision Res 1991;31: 169–187.
3. Zhou X, Qu J, Xie R, Wang R, Jiang L, Zhao H, Wen J, Lu F. Normal development of refractive state and ocular dimensions in guinea pigs. Vision Res 2006;46:2815–2823.
4. Jiang L, Schaeffel F, Zhou X, Zhang S, Jin X, Pan M, Ye L, Wu X, Huang Q, Lu F, Qu J. Spontaneous axial myopia and emmetropization in a strain of wild-type guinea pig (*Cavia porcellus*). Invest Ophthalmol Vis Sci 2009;50:1013–1019.
5. Howlett MH, McFadden SA. Emmetropization and schematic eye models in developing pigmented guinea pigs. Vision Res 2007;47:1178–1190.
6. Wang JY, Liu SZ, Wei X, Wu XY, Tan XP. High myopia and retinal ultrastructure of albino guinea-pigs. Zhong Nan Da Xue Xue Bao Yi Xue Ban 2007;32:282–287.
7. Komich RJ. Anophthalmos: an inherited trait in a new stock of guinea pigs. Am J Vet Res 1971;32:2099–2105.
8. Coster ME, Stiles J, Krohne SG, Raskin RE. Results of diagnostic ophthalmic testing in healthy guinea pigs. J Am Vet Med Assoc 2008;232:1825–1833.
9. Trost K, Skalicky M, Nell B. Schirmer tear test, phenol red thread tear test, eye blink frequency and corneal sensitivity in the guinea pig. Vet Ophthalmol 2007;10:143–146.
10. Griffith JW, Sassani JW, Bowman TA, Lang CM. Osseous choristoma of the ciliary body in guinea pigs. Vet Pathol 1988;25:100–102.
11. Kim BH, Henderson BA. Intraocular choristoma. Semin Ophthalmol 2005 20:223–229.
12. Brooks DE, McCracken MD, Collins BR. Heterotopic bone formation in the ciliary body of an aged guinea pig. Lab Anim Sci 1990;40:88–90.
13. Donnelly TM, Brown C, Donnelly TM. Heterotopic bone in the eyes of a guinea pig: osseous choristoma of the ciliary body. Lab Anim 2002;31:23–25.
14. Wu K, Kojima M, Shui YB, Sasaki H, Sasaki K. Ultraviolet B-induced corneal and lens damage in guinea pigs on low-ascorbic acid diet. Ophthalmic Res 2004;36:277–283.
15. Bettelheim FA, Churchill AC, Zigler JS Jr. On the nature of hereditary cataract in strain 13/N guinea pigs. Curr Eye Res 1997;16:917–924.
16. Racine J, Behn D, Simard E, Lachapelle P. Spontaneous occurrence of a potentially night blinding disorder in guinea pigs. Doc Ophthalmol 2003;107:59–69.

# Chapter 6

# The ferret eye

## Anatomy and physiology of the ferret eye

The ferret eye and visual system appear less well developed than in other carnivores, although it may be that the eye's diminutive size as well as its behaviour in dim light (see below) renders the ferret's vision of less importance than in related species such as the mink, which feeds more in daylight. Ferret kits are born, as are puppies and kittens, with their eyes closed but unusually, compared with the dog or cat, the eyelids do not open until as late as 28–34 days postnatally. The ferret globe is small ($7.0 \pm 0.24$ mm) [1] with a relatively large lens ($3.4 \pm 0.15$ mm) and a wide cornea for optimal light gathering in low light conditions. The animal has widely spaced laterally set (32 degrees from the midline) eyes giving a field of view of around 270 degrees but a relatively poor degree of binocularity of only about 40 degrees frontally [2]. The ovoid pupil (Figure 6.1), as with that of the cat, allows the eye a greater range of variation in admission of light from a mydriatic pupil to a tight slit, but the ferret has a horizontally orientated long axis rather than the cat's vertical pupil arrangement, presumably optimised to scan the horizon for prey items on the ground. The iris is brown in pigmented individuals (Figure 6.2) and in so-called 'black eyed white' individuals (Figure 6.2); it is not pigmented in albino animals in which the blood vessels within the iris radiate towards the pupil (Figure 6.3). Ferrets have a holangiotic fundus with retinal blood vessels radiating from the optic disc. They may appear unusually magnified on fundoscopy but this is an effect of their unusually large lens. Pigmented ferrets have a dog-like tapetum lucidum with a green–blue reflective eye-shine. Albino ferrets lack this reflectivity but are reported to have a tapetum histologically similar to that of the the pigmented wild-type ferret [3].

## What do ferrets see?

The ferret eye is optimised for function in dim and dark environments, given that in the wild the species is crepuscular, hunting its rodent prey mostly at dusk and dawn. We have little information on the visual acuity of ferrets apart from research comparing visual perception in albino and wild-type pigmented animals. On the other hand the ferret or polecat retina has been studied in detail. As we might expect from their predominantly scotopic (dim-light) vision, the ferret retina is predominantly rod-based. Research on

*Ophthalmology of Exotic Pets*, First Edition. David L. Williams.
© 2012 David Williams. Published 2012 by Blackwell Publishing Ltd.

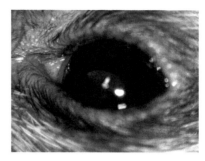

**Figure 6.1**   The normal polecat (pigmented) ferret eye with ovoid pupil.

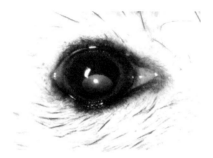

**Figure 6.2**   The 'black eyed white' ferret eye with red tapetal reflex.

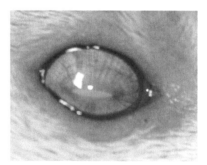

**Figure 6.3**   The albino ferret eye with red tapetal reflex.

ganglion cell density suggests that acuity is considerably lower than that of another obligate crepuscular carnivore, the cat. As with the cat, the ferret has an area of increased photoreceptor density superiotemporal to the optic disc, the area centralis. This correlates to some degree with the human macula but the ganglion cell density of the ferret is only about half that of cats, with ganglion cell receptive fields two to three times larger in the ferret than in the cat. It appears that, in terms of Snellen acuity, the ferret's visual resolution is 20/170 in bright light and 20/350 in dim light. Although the ferret's vision is markedly inferior to that of man or the cat (which is probably around 20/100), its visual sensitivity, the lower limit of light needed for vision is much better: the threshold of light needed for vision in the ferret is estimated to be five to seven times lower than in man.

As with all non-primate mammals, ferrets are dichromats, seeing with two sets of cones rather than the human three. Their peak cone density is around $26\,000/mm^2$ with a peak rod density of $350\,000/mm^2$. The ferret seems adapted to visualisation of moving objects rather than stationary ones: one study suggested that objects moving at 25–45 cm/sec were optimally visualised, perhaps correlating with the speed of rodent prey items, though this has to be said to be little more than conjecture. Other sensory agencies such as smell and hearing are important to the ferret, as may be expected in a predominantly noctural/crepuscular predator. One study suggested that olfactory cues were more important in stimulating hunting behaviour than visual ones.

We noted above that research in the ferret had for the most part been focused on the difference between pigmented and albino strains, this acting as a model for ocular abnormalities in albino animals and humans more generally. As first noted in Siamese cats, the visual fields of albino animals are substantially different from those of pigmented animals. This is certainly the case in ferrets where the far lateral retinal ganglion cells project not contralaterally, as in pigmented individuals, but ipsilaterally [4]. Defects in the optokinetic reflex in albino ferrets are also associated with defective neurogenesis and thus abnormal neurogenesis in the visual cortex [5]. This is gives rise to problems in motion detection in albino ferrets as can be shown behaviourally [6]. The same researchers measured visual acuity and contrast sensitivity in albino and normal pigmented ferrets. Interestingly they found that albino animals did not appear to have a much poorer ability in visual discrimination than their pigmented cage-mates; although there was a somewhat lower visual acuity in these albino animals it did not reach statistical significance. Females did perform less well than males in visual discrimination tests but this seemed to be a motivational rather than perceptional difference. Quite what relevance this has to pet ferrets is unclear but it may be that albino animals have poorer vision with regard to motion detection, a key feature in ferret behaviour.

# Diseases of the ferret eye

## Ophthalmia neonatorum

### Clinical signs

The late opening of the ferret kit eyelids means that infections in the conjunctival sac of kits can be severe and give rise to substantial ocular disease before being noticed. Swelling of the lids in these first weeks of the kit's life or any discharge from between the opening lids should be dealt with promptly since extension of infection can lead to panophthalmitis, subsequent septicaemia and even death. Affected kits are often anorexic, presumably because of the pain involved in the condition, but also possibly because of systemic infection spreading from the ocular region.

### Aetiopathogenesis

Ocular infection early in life can occur at birth, as seen in the cat with genital herpesvirus being passed to kittens, but in the ferret it is more commonly seen when kits suckle a jill with mastitis. Subsequent panophthalmitis and septicaemia may even result in death in severe cases [2].

### Clinical management

With regard to local treatment, the eyelids should be coaxed apart with cotton buds if near opening, or surgically if younger. Bacteriological swabs should be taken to identify the organisms involved. Topical broad-spectrum antibiotic ointment should be applied frequently. If the kits are listless or pyrexic, or the jill is shown to have an infectious mastitis, systemic antibiotics should be given to the jill and kits, although the prognosis is poor.

## Congenital ocular defects

### Clinical signs

Other congenital defects which have been reported in ferrets include microphthalmos, corneal dermoids, primary hyperplastic primary vitreous and cataracts; the latter two conditions are dealt with further below.

### Aetiopathogenesis

Microphthalmos was determined to have a simple dominant inheritance although it has to be noted that this was in one closed laboratory colony of ferrets and extrapolating this to other groups of animals may not be appropriate [7]. Corneal dermoids have been reported in ferrets and these aberrant islands of dermal tissue within the conjunctiva or cornea have in some species been determined to be inherited but in others they are sporadic defects.

### Clinical management

There is no treatment regime appropriate to resolve microphthalmos, although the persistent infection which may occur because of the over-large conjunctival sac relative to the small size of the eye may need regular management with topical antimicrobial agents. Corneal dermoids can be removed by superficial keratectomy, although the small size of the ferret eye calls for a microsurgical approach to this condition.

## Orbital disease

### Clinical signs

Space-occupying lesions in the retrobulbar space will give rise to exophthalmos with third eyelid protrusion and increased scleral 'show'. The ferret orbit is open, as is that of the dog but deeper anterior–posteriorly. This means that retrobulbar lesions are quite extensive before they are readily noted through globe protrusion anteriorly in the orbit.

### Aetiopathogenesis

Several different causes can give rise to exophthalmos from a space-occupying orbital mass. First a relatively sizeable zygomatic salivary gland fills the posterior–inferior portion of the orbit and an intraorbital salivary mucocele can develop, particularly following head trauma, given that the gland is relatively poorly encapsulated in this species [8].

Orbital neoplasia may be encountered in this species although reports are rare. Two ferrets have been reported with orbital involvement in generalised lymphoma [9].

### Clinical management

The ferret orbit has a sizeable retrobulbar venous plexus which can complicate surgical intervention in orbital disease. Nevertheless exenteration to treat orbital neoplasia has been reported in the ferret, after diagnostic imaging to determine the extent of the neoplasm [2].

## Conjunctivitis

### Clinical signs

Conjunctivitis, with the classic signs of conjunctival hyperaemia and oedema (chemosis) and an obvious mucoid to mucopurulent ocular discharge, is a relatively common finding in ferrets. These classical clinical signs of conjunctival inflammation do not allow a differentiation of the varying causes of the disease; since they are often associated with systemic disease (see below) a full clinical examination of an affected animal is mandatory.

### Aetiopathogenesis

Local irritative factors such as dusty bedding or a conjunctival foreign body can cause conjunctivitis in ferrets but in most cases the condition is a sign of systemic disease and indeed often the first sign of severe and even life-threatening conditions.

The first and most important of these is canine distemper [10]. For up to a week after exposure the ferret appears unaffected, after which a moderate to severe chemosis with mucopurulent ocular and nasal discharge is noted. The drying discharge produces brown crusting around the eyes, in severe cases leading to partial or complete fusion of the eyelids in ankyloblepharon. Blepharitis and keratoconjunctivitis sicca can also occur. Mortality rates in this condition are exceptionally high with animals dying within the first 2 weeks after infection with the ferret strain of the virus or between 3 and 5 weeks after infection with the dog strain.

Human influenza also gives rise to conjunctivitis in the ferret with initial signs very similar to those of canine distemper virus infection. The difference is that progression to severe disease with signs such as periocular crusting and ankyloblepharon do not generally occur and mortality rates are much lower [11].

Mycobacterial infection with *M. genovense* has been reported in two ferrets with proliferative conjunctivitis in one case and a more chemotic condition in the other [12]. *Salmonella* has been reported to be associated with conjunctivitis in ferrets but as a minor clinical sign in disease with other more severe characteristics such as haemorrhagic diarrhoea and pyrexia. Nutritional deficiencies, such as those associated with low dietary biotin or vitamin A, have been reported but these are likely to be rare in pet ferrets.

### Clinical management

In cases of local irritation or infection topical antibiotic preparations may be useful in cases of conjunctivitis. But since a high proportion of cases are early signs of systemic disease, a full clinical examination together with an attempt at definitive diagnosis through conjunctival swabs for polymerase chain reaction (PCR) for distemper and influenza viruses is important if the correct diagnosis and prognosis are to be given. In most cases the only treatment afforded is supportive measures and pain relief. In cases where distemper is diagnosed, many chose euthanasia as the kindest option given the high mortality rates.

In the cases of mycobacterial infection, diagnosis was by PCR investigation of material obtained by conjunctival biopsy and treatment with rifampicin together with other antibiotic medication was curative in both cases.

## Entropion

### Clinical signs

As in any species lid in-turning can give ocular discomfort and in severe cases corneal ulceration, especially if the defect is serious enough to give trichiasis with skin hair abrading onto the ocular surface (Figure 6.4).

### Aetiopathogenesis

Entropion is rare in the ferret. Anatomical abnormalities in the lid may be the cause of the condition, but in other cases an ocular surface foreign body may be responsible for initial blepharospasm which later turns into a more long-lasting defect.

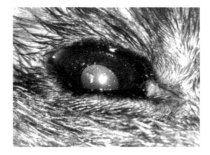

**Figure 6.4**   Lower lid entropion with trichiasis in a 6-month-old ferret.

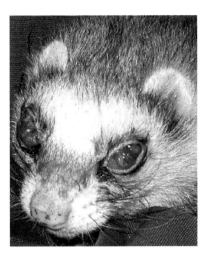

**Figure 6.5** Lymphoma presenting as third eyelid swelling and protrusion.

## Clinical management

Where ocular surface pain results from lid in-turning a foreign body should be sought by careful examination. If an anatomical defect appears to be the cause, a standard Hotz–Celsus excision of a small strip of lid skin can resolve the problem, although in a lid as small and delicate as a ferret lid, surgery under an operating microscope is to be advised.

## Adnexal lymphoma

### Clinical signs

Lymphoma is surprisingly common in the ferret but ocular manifestations are rare. One seen occasionally is lymphomatous enlargement of the tissue on the bulbar surface of the third eyelid (Figure 6.5).

### Aetiopathogenesis

Quite why lymphoma appears so common in the older ferret is unclear but one large survey suggested that in reality the incidence of neoplasia is not higher than in the dog or cat [13], while another study showed that a high proportion were T cell neoplasms with related poor prognosis [14].

### Clinical management

While various chemotherapeutic regimes have been reported for lymphoma in the ferret, in this author's experience these neoplasms when involving the eyes are refractory to treatment. Topical steroid can reduce the inflammatory reaction for a time and topical tear replacement similarly eases ocular surface discomfort.

### *Keratitis*

#### *Clinical signs*

Corneal disease in the ferret may be usefully categorised into ulcerative and non-ulcerative keratitis. Corneal ulcers can be evaluated as in any other species by use of fluorescein dye to determine when epithelial integrity has been lost. Non-ulcerative keratitis may be characterised by vascularisation and a cellular infiltrate.

#### *Aetiopathogenesis*

Corneal ulceration may be associated with trauma, tear deficiency or exposure keratitis. Epithelial basement membrane dystrophy, as seen in dogs and rabbits, has not been reported in ferrets, but in older animals delayed epithelial healing can give rise to similar signs. Tear production in ferrets has been documented at $5.3 \pm 1.3$ mm/min using a standard Schirmer tear test strip, giving a useful guide suggesting when tear deficiency may be involved in corneal disease. Assessment should also be made of the degree of exposure of the central cornea since corneal ulceration may be associated with exposure keratitis, as reported in a ferret with exophthalmos from a salivary mucocele [2].

The non-ulcerative keratitis may be immune-mediated in origin as in canine chronic superficial keratitis, but it has also been reported as an early sign of multicentric lymphoma in one ferret [15].

#### *Clinical management*

Corneal ulceration should be managed as in other species with topical antibiosis alone if traumatic in origin or with topical cyclosporine ointment (Optimmune, Schering-Plough) and tear replacement (a carbomer gel such as Viscotears, Allergan) if associated with keratoconjunctivitis sicca. If exposure keratitis is a causative factor, clearly amelioration of the cause of the globe protrusion is essential but if this is not possible in the short term, a lateral canthoplasty will reduce the degree of exposure until resolution of the corneal exposure is achieved.

### *Uveitis*

#### *Clinical signs*

The classic signs of miosis, episcleral hyperaemia and frank signs of intraocular inflammation such as keratic precipitates and hypopyon may be missed initially because of the small size of the ferret eye, but pain and photophobia should encourage further examination of an inflamed eye in a ferret as with any other species. The predominant sign seen by this author is corneal oedema (Figure 6.6), with uveitis differentiated from glaucoma by the fact that the inflamed eyes have a lower intraocular pressure than those with glaucoma.

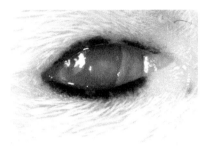

**Figure 6.6**  Uvetitis with corneal oedema and an intraocular pressure of 8 mmHg.

### Aetiopathogenesis

Uveitis is not a commonly reported condition in the ferret and most cases involve break-down of the blood–aqueous barrier secondary to trauma or corneal ulceration. The one condition in which uveitis is an important primary sign is Aleutian disease, a generalised parvoviral immune complex disease. Mink experimentally infected with the virus developed a significant anterior and intermediate uveitis involving the iris and ciliary body predominantly; this has also been reported in a naturally infected otter. While ferrets with the disease have not been specifically reported with uveitis this may well be through inattention to ocular signs given that vasculitis is a classical feature of the disease and inflammation of uveal vasculature classically causes a breakdown in the blood–aqueous barrier with subsequent uveitis. Other causes of uveitis in ferrets may include systemic fungal diseases, such as blastomycosis and cryptococcosis, and protozoal diseases, such as toxoplasmosis.

### Clinical management

Use of atropine as a mydriatic and cycloplegic is important in anterior uveitis but the small size of the ferret eye and the small blood volume means that over-exuberant medication with this parasympatholytic could result in systemic toxicity. As uveitis may be an early sign of systemic disease in the ferret, any animal with intraocular inflammation should be subject to a full clinical examination and blood work-up.

### Cataract

### Clinical signs

Lens opacification starting as small cortical vacuoles or spokes and progressing to full milky white cataract is surprisingly common in some reports of ferrets from laboratory environments although, in this author's experience, it is less common in outbred ferrets kept as pets. Most are seen in older ferrets over 5 years of age in which lens opacification is more common. Nuclear sclerosis occurs in middle-aged ferrets prior to frank opacification. Close examination of the ferret eye with either direct or indirect ophthalmoscopy will show opacities in the lens capsule, cortex or nucleus. Early focal opacities appear

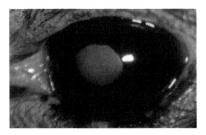

**Figure 6.7**   Diffuse maturing cataract in an 8-year-old ferret.

predominantly as pinpoint reflections of light, while mature cataract is seen as a diffuse haze or more profound opacity similar to those in other species (Figure 6.7).

### Aetiopathogenesis

In one report 47% of year-old ferrets had some degree of lens opacity ranging from punctate opacities to hypermature cataracts, while by 18 months of age almost all ferrets in the colony had some degree of cataract [16]. Another report, already noted above, documented microphthalmia with congenital cataract in a group of inbred laboratory ferrets [7,17]. A study ongoing by our group has found age-related nuclear sclerosis in ferrets over 4 years of age while 50% of the population have frank focal opacities as the beginning of age-related cataract by the age of 5 years. By the age of 7 years all ferrets have some degree of age-related cataract formation.

### Clinical management

Removal of a cataractous ferret lens is difficult given the small size of the ferret globe. Irrigation–aspiration is more likely to be successful than phacoemulsification given the size of the probes involved, although most animals are not overly affected by the mild lens opacification occurring in middle to old age, and so probably do not require any surgery.

### Lens luxation

### Clinical signs

Lens luxations are readily noted in the ferret eye by assessment of the aphakic crescent which occurs as the lens first subluxates out of the visual axis of the globe. Many are associated with mature cataract and thus movement of the lens is particularly easily appreciated, either forward into the anterior chamber or backwards, falling in to the vitreous cavity. Intraocular pressure should be determined with a hand-held applanation or rebound tonometer; often intraocular pressure is raised because of impairment of aqueous outflow by the large lens sitting in the anterior chamber or by vitreous strands blocking the iridocorneal angle. At other times intraocular pressure may be reduced, presumably as a result of mild intraocular inflammation, although concurrent signs of uveitis are not generally present.

### Aetiopathogenesis

Most lens luxations in ferrets occur because of cataract formation within the lens which puts tension on the lens zonule but primary luxations have also been noted.

### Clinical management

Removal of the lens by irrigation–aspiration or by intracapsular lendectomy may be attempted but the small size of the ferret eye renders the surgery more difficult and in this author's experience, where the animal is not inconvenienced by the luxation, cases may be better managed by conservative medical therapy to reduce intraocular pressure (see below) or control mild inflammation.

## Glaucoma

### Clinical signs

Glaucoma is an uncommon condition in the ferret. Episcleral injection, mydriasis and blindness are signs of raised intraocular pressure in the ferret as with other species. The normal intraocular pressure in the ferret has been reported as $22.8 \pm 5.5$ mmHg in one study using rhe Tonopen applanation tonometer [18] and $21.0 \pm 4.0$ mmHg in another study using anaesthetised ferrets; a third study determined the intraocular pressure to be considerably lower at $14.5 \pm 3.2$ mmHg. Recent measurements on 80 normal ferrets from this author's clinic using the Tonovet rebound tonometer determined the normal intraocular pressure to be $13.1 \pm 1.1$ mmHg.

### Aetiopathogenesis

No cases of primary glaucoma have been reported in the veterinary literature and all cases seen in the author's clinic have been secondary to uveitis after trauma or luxation of cataractous lenses.

### Clinical management

Medical management of glaucoma in ferrets with topical dorzolamide, pilocarpine or the prostaglandin analogue latanoprost has been reported [19], although no data were given with regard to efficacy of these drugs; this quite understandable given the rarity of the conditon in this species. The same review reported the successful use of trans-scleral diode laser cytophotocoagulation to control raised intraocular pressure in one ferret.

## Retinal disease

### Clinical signs

Retinal degeneration in ferrets has been reported to be common [20] with signs of tapetal hyper-reflectivity and vascular attenuation as one might find in a dog or cat with inherited degeneration seen in progressive retinal atrophy.

### Aetiopathogenesis

While some suggest a familial trait in such degeneration, the fact that the ferret, like the cat, is an obligate carnivore, suggests that, as in what used to be called feline central retinal degeneration, dietary taurine deficiency may play a part in the retinal atrophy. Were this to be the case one might expect to see early changes in the area centralis, as occurs in the cat, but to date none has been reported in the literature.

Intrauterine infection with feline panleucopenia virus has been shown to cause a widespread devastating retinopathy with subsequent blindness, but this infection has not been reported occurring naturally [21].

### Clinical management

Without a clear aetiology for these blinding retinopathies in the ferret little can be offered in advice regarding treatment or prevention except to say that, given their often nocturnal habits in the wild, many ferrets appear to cope well with blindness and that owners should not be unduly perturbed if their pet is found to be visually impaired.

## References

1. Hernández-Guerra AM, Rodilla V, López-Murcia MM. Ocular biometry in the adult anesthe-tized ferret (*Mustela putorius furo*). Vet Ophthalmol 2007;10:50–52.
2. Miller PE. Ferret ophthalmology. Sem Avian Exotic Pet Med 1997;6:146–151.
3. Tjalve H, Frank A. Tapetum lucidum in the pigmented and albino ferret. Exp Eye Res 1984;38:341–351.
4. Garipis N, Hoffmann KP. Visual field defects in albino ferrets (*Mustela putorius furo*). Vsion Res 2003;3:793–800.
5. Hoffmann KP, Garipis N, Distler C. *Optokinetic deficits in albino ferrets (Mustela putorius furo)*: a behavioral and electrophysiological study. J Neurosci 2004;24:4061–4069.
6. Hupfeld D, Distler C, Hoffmann KP. Motion perception deficits in albino ferrets (*Mustela putorius furo*). Vision Res 2006;46:2941–2948.
7. Miler PE, Dubielzig RR. Autosomal dominant microphthalmia, cataract and retinal dysplasia in a laboratory colony of ferrets. Invest Ohthalmol Vis Sci 1995;36:S64.
8. Miller PE, Pickett JP. Zygomatic salivary mucocele in a ferret. J Am Vet Med Assoc 1989;184:1437–1438.
9. McCalla TL, Erdman SE, Kawasaki T. Lymphoma with orbital involvement in two ferrets. Prog Vet Comp Ophthalmol 1997;7:36–38.
10. Davidson MG. Canine distemper virus infection in the domestic ferret. Comp Cont Educ 1986;8:448–453.
11. Ryland LM, Gorham JR. The ferret and its diseases. J Am Vet Med Assoc 1978;173: 1154–1158.
12. Lucas J, Lucas A, Furber H, James G, Hughes MS, Martin P, Chen SC, Mitchell DH, Love DN, Malik R. Mycobacterium genavense infection in two aged ferrets with conjunctival lesions. Aust Vet J 2000;78:685–689.
13. Li X, Fox JG, Padrid PA. Neoplastic diseases in ferrets: 574 cases (1968–1997). J Am Vet Med Assoc 1998;212:1402–1406.

14. Onuma M, Kondo H, Ono S, Shibuya H, Sato T. Cytomorphological and immunohistochemical features of lymphoma in ferrets. J Vet Med Sci 2008;70:893–898

15. Ringle MJ, Lindley DM, Krohne SG. Lymphoplasmacytic keratitis in a ferret with lymphoma. J Am Vet Med Assoc 1993;203:670–672.

16. Miller PE, Marler AJ, Dubielzig RR. Cataracts in a laboratory colony of ferrets. Lab Anim Sci 1993;43:562–568.

17. Miller PE, Dubielzig RR. The morphology of autosomal dominant microphthalmia in ferrets. 26th ACVO Congress 1995:62.

18. Sapienza JS, Procher D, Collins BR. Tonometry in clinically normal ferrets. Prog Vet Comp Ophthalmol 1991;1:291–294.

19. Good KL. Ocular disorders in pet ferrets. Vet Clin N Am 2002;5:325–339.

20. Kawasaki T. Retinal atrophy in the ferret. J Sm Exotic Anim Med 1992;1:137.

21. Margolis G, Kilham L. Retinopathy in experimental prenatal and early postnatal infections with reovirus 3, mumps virus and feline panleucopaenia virus. J Neuropathol Exp Neurol 1974;3:178.

# Chapter 7

# The rat and mouse eye

We will cover the rat and mouse eye together; although they have some differences in basic biology and disease, for the most part the same sort of conditions are seen in both and their overall anatomy and physiology are similar. I have previously reviewed ocular conditions in the rat [1], and Richard Smith's masterful monograph gives all the information one could need for, as its title suggests, the mouse eye [2].

## Anatomy of the eye

The small size of the laboratory rodent eye renders close ophthalmic examination somewhat difficult without practice. Having said that, nocturnal species often have comparatively bigger eyes than diurnal animals, but with most rodents being adapted for night vision the eyes are relatively small and, though it pains me as a comparative ophthalmologist to say this, vision is relatively less important to these rodents than to many other species.

Rats and mice have three lacrimal structures, the intraorbital gland, situated deep in the orbit, the extraorbital gland, located near the base of the masseter muscle, and the Harderian gland positioned as a U shape around the optic nerve behind the globe [3].

The cornea is very thin in these species and the lens is spherical, taking up a large amount of the intraocular volume, in order to focus light on the retina in such a small eye. Almost all rodents have a round pupil, but chinchillas have a slit pupil somewhat like that of a cat. Albino rodents have a non-pigmented iris with a red reflex and little opportunity to reduce illumination falling on the retina. This is important when considering reasons for phototoxicity in animals kept in too light an environment, whether at home or in the laboratory.

While the iris of albino animals rarely needs dilating, and does so rapidly if tropicamide is applied, the irides of pigmented rats and mice can be taxing to widen. They resist the pharmacological dilation provided normally by topical atropine, probably because melanin binds atropine, reducing the drug availability at the motor end plate of the parasympathetic nerve. 1% atropine followed by 10% phenylephrine every five minutes rapidly provides adequate pupil dilation, although toxic effects of systemically absorbed drugs should be watched for. Retinal phototoxicity has been noted in bright light after mydriasis so ambient light should be reduced in animals after pupil dilation [4].

*Ophthalmology of Exotic Pets*, First Edition. David L. Williams.
© 2012 David Williams. Published 2012 by Blackwell Publishing Ltd.

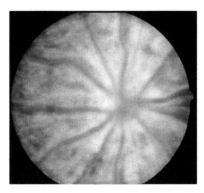

**Figure 7.1**  The holangiotic retina of a pigmented rat eye.

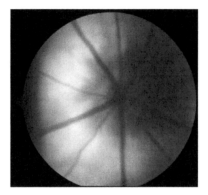

**Figure 7.2**  The holangiotic retina of an albino mouse eye.

Rats have an orbital venous plexus which is important to note when performing an enucleation [5]. While mice may be at a lower risk of haemorrhage during this operation, their small size means that even limited blood loss during enucleation should be avoided at all costs [6].

The fundus of the rat and mouse is holangiotic with retinal venules and arterioles radiating from the optic nerve head. The choroid underlying these vessels is pigmented in pigmented strains (Figure 7.1) but devoid of pigment in albinos (Figure 7.2).

## A note on ophthalmoscopy

As noted in the introductory chapter on examination techniques, the small size of rat and particularly mouse eyes, renders fundoscopy somewhat taxing. Indirect ophthalmoscopy with +30–40 D can be useful since the large lens tends to distort the view of the fundus by direct ophthalmoscopy. A particularly useful method of observing and recording the fundus in small rodents is to use an operating microscope with the rodent under a general anaesthetic which dilates the pupil, and the highly convex cornea covered with one drop of viscous solution (2% methylcellulose for instance) held in place with a flat cover slip over the eye. The animal's eye can then be observed with an operating microscrope.

Another useful technique is to use a drop of similar viscous fluid between the cornea and a rigid endoscope which allows ready viewing of the entire fundus; recording is also possible if a photographic attachment is added [7].

Tear film evaluation with the Schirmer tear test is impractical in these species because of the large size of the filter paper strip. The phenol red thread test is to be preferred, although we do not have detailed normal ranges for tear production in most laboratory species [8]. Tonometry is difficult in rats and next to impossible in the mouse with the Tonopen applanation tonometer because of its sizeable footplate compared to the ocular surface diameter in these species. The Tonovet or Tonolab, a rebound tonometer, is much more appropriate for these species since its rebounding probe takes up less than $1\,mm^2$ of cornea [9].

## What do rats and mice see?

Being by nature nocturnal animals, the rat (*Rattus novergicus*) and the mouse (*Mus musculus*) have rod-dominated retinas but with cones containing visual pigments that absorb with a peak sensitivity at 359 nm with 'blue-UV' cones and at 510 nm with middle 'green' cones [10,11]. About 88% of a rat's cones are the middle green type, and 12% are the blue-UV cones, these mostly located in a zone in the ventral retina [12]. The ultraviolet sensitivity is important in two ways – at dawn and dusk the ratio of ultraviolet wavelengths compared with those of visible light is higher and thus a UV sensitivity may give a significant advantage in these crepuscular species.

Rat visual acuity is relatively poor, as might be expected from their relative deficiency in cone photoreceptors. Human visual acuity is around 30 cycles per degree (cpd) while that of a normal pigmented rat is reported as 1 cpd, and 0.5 cpd for albino rats in one study [13]; another report gives values of 1.2 cpd for pigmented rats and 0.34–0.43 cpd for albino rats [14]. Such measurements suggest that a normally pigmented rat has about 20/600 vision, while albino rats have about 20/1200 vision. If rat acuity is measured by determining ganglion cell density of ganglion cells in the retina, the area of maximum ganglion cell density is 52.8 degrees wide, this being above and temporal to the optic disc with a maximum density at $6774$ cells/mm$^2$ compared with the human fovea with a density of $38\,000$ cells/mm$^2$ [15]. This ganglion cell density suggests a maximum visual acuity of 1.5 cpd, which is consistent with the values from photoreceptor density and also from behavioral acuity experiments [16]. Having said that, acuity can be influenced by many factors, especially during development, as Hubert and Weissel showed in their seminal Nobel prize-winning studies on cats [17]. Rodent visual acuity is significantly improved by environmental enrichment [18], but visual deprivation, on the other hand, causes substantial decreases in visual acuity in both juvenile rats [19] and mice [20], paralleling the changes seen in high mammals such as primates and man. Interestingly though, visual deprivation can lead to increases in visual acuity in rats [21] and mice [22].

The very lateral placement of the rat eyes (Figure 7.3) renders their depth perception by binocular vision defective. This ocular positioning gives this prey species a wide field of view, with their field of binocular vision being only about 76 degrees, while that of humans is around 105 degrees [10]. Rats rely on motion parallax rather than binocular

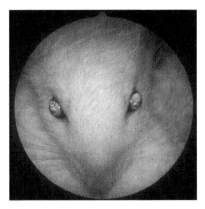

**Figure 7.3** The protuberant eyes of an albino rat.

vision to estimate depth, with vertical head bobs allowing them to judge distance. An experiment requiring rats to jump between two platforms showed a greater number and more pronounced head bobs before jumping as the gap between platforms increased [23].

Albino rats and mice have lower visual acuity than pigmented individuals, as noted above, this being due to a number of factors. Photoreceptor development requires dopa, a molecule derived through the action of tyrosinase, the enzyme deficient in albino animals. Thus the albino rat or mouse retina has around 30% fewer photoreceptors than its pigmented compatriot [24] and the rods it does have are relatively depleted of rhodopsin [25]. The lack of melanin also makes dark adaptation slower in albino animals; pigmented rats adapt to the dark in around 30 minutes, but albino rats are reported to take six times as long [26]. Such a deficit may be important in laboratories where lights are switched on and off with regularity. Perhaps a more worrying effect on albino rodents of living in a relatively well lit environment such as a research laboratory, is that light toxicity is all too common where miosis has no effect on the amount of light reaching the retina, as is the case in animals with albinoid irides. The light levels required by UK Home Office regulations of research establishments in the UK are limited to 350–400 lux. Given the lack of detection of wavelengths at the red end of the visible light spectrum, the use of red plastic hide boxes in such housing prevents this retinal degeneration and allows animals to behave as if they were in the dark, while allowing animal technicians to evaluate the animals with acceptable illumination.

## Ophthalmic disease in rats and mice

### *Chromodacryorrhoea*

#### *Clinical signs*

Rodents with chromodacryorrhoea exhibit red staining or crusting around their eyes (Figure 7.4), and sometimes near the nostrils and also on the dorsal surface of their front feet, as they have rubbed their periocular regions [27].

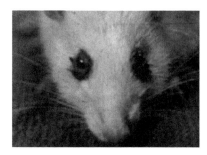

**Figure 7.4**   Chromodacryorrhoea in a stressed rat. (Reproduced courtesy of Dr L. Bauck.)

## Aetiopathology

The lacrimal glands of rodents such as the rat and mouse differ quite substantially from those of companion animal species, and one of the main ways in which this is manifest is their production of porphyrin pigments in the tears at times of stress. This so-called chromodacryorrhoea occurs during parasympathetic stimulation of the Harderian gland, one of the orbital glands involved in tear production. This periocular red staining or crusting can be seen as a feature of diseases such as mycoplasmosis or sialodacryoad-enitis but also during periods of stress such as restraint, rehousing with unfamiliar animals or transport. Harderian gland swelling and necrosis have been reported after aberrant exposure of rats to excessive levels of light and it may well be that these patho-logical changes were caused by the deleterious photodynamic effects of light on the Harderian gland and its porphyrin products [28].

## Clinical management

The key feature in the management of chromodacryorrhoea is finding and resolving the stressors which have led to the condition. Until these are ameliorated one cannot hope to control the condition and the impeded welfare which it signals. In an individ-ual animal topical tear replacement can be helpful in ameliorating associated ocular discomfort.

## Ocular surface trauma

### Clinical signs

The relatively large size of the ocular surface in these species compared to the globe volume, and the prominence of the eye renders these animals prone to ocular surface trauma (Figure 7.5). This is particularly true given the environments in which they are often kept with sawdust or hay shards all too frequently agents of tramautic injury. Corneal ulceration can be visualised in these species as in others, with the use of a small drop of fluorescein rapidly flushed away with a stream of sterile water or normal saline solution. Ocular discharge may be seen with surface trauma or with intraorbital disease as noted further below. It is important to differentiate these two mechanisms of ocular

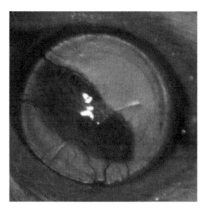

**Figure 7.5**  Vascularised corneal ulcer in a rat after ocular surface exposure following a ketamine/xylazine anaesthetic.

injury. Intraorbital infection gives exophthalmos, blepharitis and epiphora with or without discharge as well as hemifacial swelling, although these signs are seen less commonly in the rat and mouse than in the chinchilla or hamster.

### Aetiopathology

As noted above traumatic injury may be seen relatively regularly in small rodents, if owners or carers are careful enough to observe it. The same can be said of intraorbital disease secondary to tooth root abscessation which can be seen in any rodent species. While surface trauma occurs after direct interaction with an environmental insult, intraorbital space-occupying lesions such as abscesses cause exophthalmos which can readily result in surface trauma, thus potentially making the differentiation of these two somewhat difficult at times.

### Clinical management

Topical antibiotic is worthwhile applying to surface post-traumatic lesions to avoid secondary bacterial infection. Ocular lubrication with a carbomer-based gel or a hypromellose drop can similarly reduce irritation and inflammation, as well as speeding corneal epithelial healing.

## Conjunctivitis and systemic disease

### Clinical signs

Conjunctivitis in laboratory rodents may be manifest in a number of different forms from excess clear tearing through to a frank purulent discharge with profound conjunctival hyperaemia.

## Aetiopathogenesis

Conjunctivitis in rats and mice may be caused by local irritative agents such as dusty bedding. It should be noted that it can often be a sign of upper respiratory disease caused by *Mycoplasma* or less commonly other agents such as viruses or bacteria, regularly compounded by poor ventilation [29]. The presence of one aetiological factor does not rule out the involvement of others – the possible involvement of *Mycoplasma* together with dusty bedding borne on air currents caused by deficient ventilation underlines the potential multifactorial nature of this disease. An outbreak of conjunctivitis in laboratory rodents is therefore to be investigated thoroughly with attention paid to affected animal, cage-mates and the environment in which they are housed.

The genetic background of the animals has also to be taken into account: athymic nu/nu mice lack eyelashes and forelimb hair preventing them from removing particulate matter from their ocular surface. In these animals their deficiency immune status also renders them susceptible to colonisation by microorganisms.

## Clinical management

Clearly management of these cases depends on a thorough investigation of the factors which may be important in their genesis. Correction of deficiences in the environment may be a long-term project, but is central to optimising the welfare of the animals, whether they be a child's pet or a colony of research animals; it will also ensure that the results obtained from research on the animals in this second example are acceptable from a scientific perspective. Investigating the animals themselves should include close ophthalmoscopic or slit lamp examination to determine if there is purely conjunctivitis, or conjunctivitis with a concurrent keratitis. Samples should be taken for bacteriology and polymerase chain reaction (PCR) for *Mycoplasma*, unless it is already known that a chronic subclinical infectious problem exists. In such a case it is important to look for additional factors exacerbating the underlying problem. These could range from the stress caused by a new member of staff handling the animals to a novel research procedure or change in the environment precipitating additional conjunctival pathology.

It must be appreciated that once an outbreak of conjunctivitis occurs, especially if it is associated with upper respiratory infection, it can be very difficult to eradicate. Complete depopulation may be required if the situation is severe with deleterious effects on animal welfare or research validity. A vicious circle can be promoted in which conjunctivitis and upper respiratory infection exacerbate stress which further worsens the animals' ocular condition.

## Sialodacryoadenitis virus

### Clinical signs

This condition, previously described as the most devastating adnexal disease of rats, starts as an episode of blepharospasm, photophobia and ocular irritation manifested as continual eye rubbing [30]. After initiation excess lacrimation, tear gland hyperplasia and subsequent necrosis lead to a severe reduction in tear production. Keratitis, conjunctivitis and periocular swelling occur partly through tear deficiency but more probably directly related to self-mutilation [31]. Chromodacryorrhoea (see above) is a common sequel, through this trauma and associated stress. Sometimes intraocular inflammation and secondary glaucoma can occur. The disease itself is self-limiting with improvement within 1 week, but the secondary signs may take more than a month to resolve if they do completely.

### Aetiopathogenesis

Sialodacryoadenitis is caused by a coronavirus, first described in 1961, but given that the disease signs occur as a result of the interaction between the virus and the host immune system, the exact nature, severity and duration of the disease varies between strains and is influenced by external factors and internal influences such as degree of stress and the immune status of the animals [32]. Studies on immunosuppressed rats showed that experimentally impeding the immune response to the virus with cyclophosphamide delayed the onset of signs, reduced the severity of gland damage but led to a lengthening of the disease and also persistent viral shedding [33]. Repair processes which naturally occur in infected glands involve squamous metaplasia of duct epithelium with potential reduction in tearing.

### Clinical management

The disease is often diagnosed by its pathognomonic signs, but detection of anticorona-viral antibodies is possible. Such serological testing has shown that up to 45% of colonies within the United Kingdom have been exposed to the virus, although incidence of overt disease is significantly lower [34]. This finding highlights the potential danger of adding a set of naïve animals into a subclinically affected colony which may provoke onset of overt clinical disease. Individual animals should be managed with tear replacement gel to counteract the deleterious effects of lacrimal insufficiency.

## Microphthalmos and anophthalmos

### Clinical signs

The occurrence of pathologically small eyes in laboratory rodents, or in severe cases the absence of an eye altogether, is a not uncommon condition in certain strains of laboratory rodents and thus also in some pet mice, given the large numbers of laboratory animals which find their way into pet shops. Microphthalmic eyes often have abnormal iridal vasculature (Figure 7.6), but the most obvious sign is a sunken small globe in a relatively large orbit, sometimes with associated ocular discharge.

### Aetiopathogenesis

Absence of ocular tissue, or small size of the eye, can be seen as an inherited trait in laboratory rodents [35]. This is particularly the case in C57 black mice where microphthalmos is a regular occurrence [36]. It has been suggested by some workers that this abnormality in globe development is associated with a defective lens morphology [37].

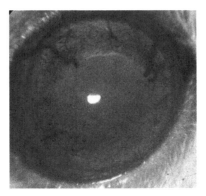

**Figure 7.6** Iris vascular congestion in a microphthalmic mouse eye. (Reproduced courtesy of Mr Peter Lee.)

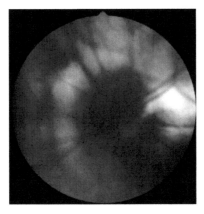

**Figure 7.7** Persistent hyaloid vasculature with haemorrhage in a 6-week-old rat. (Reproduced courtesy of Mr Peter Lee.)

### Clinical management

Clearly a congenital small eye cannot be cured but the key feature causing problems is infection in the relatively large orbit. Topical antibiotic medication is valuable to resolve such problems and may be useful prophylactically to prevent chronic orbital infection.

### Persistent embryological vasculature

### Clinical signs

Persistence of the hyaloid artery is a common finding in rats and mice (Figure 7.7). In one study of ICR and BALB/c mice, 28% of the former and 32% of the latter strains had persistent hyaloid vasculature appearing as a white strand in the vitreous, with 100% of animals aged up to 2 weeks having the condition, reducing to 43% by 11 weeks. The more concerning finding is vitreal haemorrhage associated with this persistent vasculature.

## Aetiopathogenesis

Congenital persistence of the hyaloid vasculature may be an inherited trait but a specific gene mutation has not been identified.

## Clinical management

No treatment is successful in such cases nor required since, although the posterior segment haemorrhage may obscure vision and on occasion led to uveitis or increased intraocular pressure, such sequelae are rare.

## Non-ulcerative corneal lesions

## Clinical signs

Corneal opacification may be related to keratitis, to lipid stromal dystrophy or to subepithelial calcification or indeed to a mixture of these different pathologies. Some cases, such as dystrophic change in CD1 mice, are characterised by a central white oval lesion (Figure 7.8); other cases, such as corneal calcification, show a more general white heterogeneous scarring. Where inflammation supervenes the lesion can become predominantly vascularised. In their study of ICR and BALB/c mice, Park and colleagues noted around 4% of animals from both strains with corneal scars, most probably traumatic in origin [38]. Heywood noted that many similar lesions in rats have associated concurrent secondary uveitis [39], (see further below).

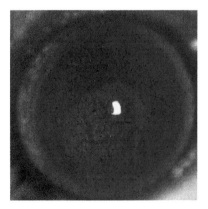

**Figure 7.8**  Corneal dystrophy in a CD-1 mouse.

### Aetiopathogenesis

Corneal lesions can have a number of aetiologies in rodents and elucidating which is important in a specific case can be difficult. Nasal corneal opacities are relatively common in laboratory rodents and can be a sequel to orbital gland inflammation or intraocular inflammation, or can exist as an ocular surface disorder alone. There may well be an association with reduced tear secretion or with environmental changes such as increased ammonia in the microenvironment of the cage floor area.

Mineral deposits in the superficial subepithelial stroma have been noted on histopathological examination of these eyes; in some cases inflammation supervenes, while in others mineralization is the only change. Dietary deficiencies in nutrients such as vitamin A have, in the past, been reported as causes of such pathology, but the nutritional adequacy of diets for laboratory or pet rodents these days makes such factors less likely to play a part in corneal disease.

### Clinical management

In animals where keratitis is noted, a thorough investigation of the environment and microenvironment should be undertaken to ensure that increased levels of ammonia or other noxious agents are not instrumental in the genesis of corneal pathology.

## Corneal ulcers

### Clinical signs

Ulcerative keratitis in rats and mice can be delineated with the use of a small drop of fluorescein dye followed by flushing of the ocular surface. Most ulcers are superficial although some can progress deeper into the stroma. Depth can be assessed by visualising the reflection of incident light from the corneal surface adjacent to the ulcer and the reflection from the centre of the ulcer. In superficial ulceration there is little gap between the two, while in a deep ulcer the two reflections are separated from each other by the depth of the ulcer.

Animals with epithelial defects alone will present with an irritated eye with an area of epithelial erosion, positive with fluorescein dye but with no other signs of corneal disease. Deeper stromal ulcers generally also manifest with a variable degree of corneal oedema but a relatively crisp ulcer boundary. Any ulcer in which this defined margin appears blurred or irregular may be developing into a melting ulcer or stromal abscess and should be observed carefully. Many of these more serious ulcers will also give rise to an anterior uveitis with a miotic pupil, aqueous flare (which can be difficult at times to differentiate from the corneal haze also present) and sometimes frank inflammatory debris in the manner of hypopyon.

Stromal abscessation describes the situation where infectious organisms and associated purulent material, often resulting from a corneal injury, are trapped in the stroma by re-epithelialisation. Thus the cornea does not stain with fluorescein dye but may be infiltrated by new blood vessels or further stromal inflammatory cell populations. Uveitis with flare and miosis often accompanies such signs.

## Aetiopathogenesis

Corneal ulcers in these rodents are often post-traumatic in origin with or without an infectious organism also supervening. Epithelial defects generally heal rapidly while stromal ulcers may be refractory to healing, especially where there is also an infectious organism involved. Indeed this rapid epithelialisation can be a problem where it covers and traps infectious material giving a stromal abscess.

## Clinical management

Most corneal ulcers in these animals will heal spontaneously, but the likelihood of complication by infectious organisms means that topical antibiosis with a broad-spectrum antibiotic ointment should be standard practice. Given the prevalence of Gram-negative organisms the choice of topical antibiotic should be chloramphenicol, a fluoroquinolone such as ofloxacin or ciprofloxacin, or gentamicin; fusidic acid is not recommended as it only has antibiotic activity against Gram-positive cocci.

Where uveitis is evident, as manifest by miosis or flare, one atropine drop or atropine ointment should be applied. The small size of these animals means that the transconjunctival uptake of such medications can give the problem of systemic toxicity. The use of one drop alone, or indeed of ointments which limit systemic uptake and prolong drug availability in the precorneal tear film should be emphasised to owners to avoid the overuse of topical medication in these small animals.

In some cases of severe stromal abscessation, surgical removal of infectious material may be attempted, but the very thin nature of the cornea in these rodents, and particularly mice, renders such surgery hazardous and it should only be undertakien under an operating microscope. As such, surgery for an individual rat or mouse pet is generally not financially viable, nor particularly beneficial for the welfare of the animal. Similarly culture and sensitivity evaluation for bacteriological samples is generally not appropriate in individual animals but a Gram stain and modified Giemsa stain of a corneal sample will allow one to tell whether Gram-positive cocci or Gram-negative rods are involved, or maybe that the condition is fungal in origin.

## Exposure keratopathy

## Clinical signs

Corneal surface pathology, which may be ulcerative or non-ulcerative, may be seen either after anaesthetic or when the globe is abnormally protruding, either through enlargement in glaucoma or proptosis through a retrobulbar space-occupying mass. The lesion is more often than not vascularised if chronic and may or may not be ulcerated (see Figure 7.5).

## Aetiopathogenesis

Exposure keratopathy can occur especially during and after anaesthesia if eyelids are not taped closed during a prolonged procedure. This is particularly the case in animals anaesthetised with a xylazine/ketamine regime; it is particularly noted in Wistar, Long Evans and Fischer 344 strains more than in Sprague-Dawley and Lewis rats, suggesting that there is a genetic component to the predisposition for such changes as well as a drug-related agency. Other reasons include ocular surface exposure through globe enlargement often seen in glaucoma (see below) or with a retrobulbar space-occupying mass, either a neoplasm or abscess.

### Clinical management

As noted above, anaesthetised animals should have their eyes taped shut during an procedure or have a lubricant such as the carbomer-based Viscotears or lanolin-based Lacrilube applied to prevent exposure keratitis. In animals with proptosis ocular surface lubrication can reduce the likelihood of severe ocular surface damage, although management of the underlying problem, if possible, is obviously to be recommended.

## Congenital abnormalities of the uvea

### Clinical signs

Colobomas or absence of tissue, may be observed at the 6 o'clock position in some mouse strains (Figure 7.9). Such a sign must be differentiated from a synechia, where an inflamed iris has adhered to the anterior lens capsule (Figure 7.10). This can be difficult but in the absence of other signs of intraocular inflammation such as miosis or flare, and especially if several related animals are affected with otherwise quiet eyes, a ventral coloboma can be diagnosed.

### Aetiopathogenesis

Colobomas can be inherited or occur during intrauterine development because of maternal disease, often with pyrexia, during gestation. In the case of a 6 o'clock coloboma the

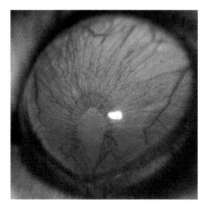

**Figure 7.9**  A typical (6 o'clock) coloboma in a CD-1 mouse. (Reproduced courtesy of Mr Peter Lee.)

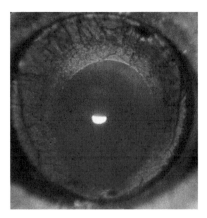

**Figure 7.10**  Ventral synechia in a Wistar rat with uveitis.

lesion has occurred because of defective fusion of the optic cup in which the ventral optic fissure does not close adequately.

### Clinical management

There is generally no need for treatment in such cases but the presence of an incidental coloboma in a toxicity study, for instance, should not be taken as a drug effect, but more likely a spontaneous incidental finding.

### Uveitis

### Clinical signs

Intraocular inflammation is not commonly seen in rats and mice but, on the other hand, is not vanishingly rare. The classic triad of miosis, blepharospasm and photophobia together with evidence of anterior chamber inflammatory debris should be sufficient to give a firm diagnosis where present. Note however that haemorrhage in the anterior or posterior chambers is not sufficient evidence to lead to a diagnosis since persistence of the tunica vasculosa lentis, which supplies the lens with nutrition in utero, or the hyaloid vasculature in the posterior chamber can lead to intraocular haemorrhage without inflammation (Figure 7.11). On the other hand intraocular inflammation in these rodents can be manifest by iridal hyperaemia alone, as seen in Figure 7.10, and does not always manifest as overt inflammatory deposits as with the hypopyon seen in cat and dogs.

### Aetiopathogenesis

A number of experimental manipulations can give rise to uveitis in rodents held in research but we have little understanding of what causes uveitis in pet rats or mice. Thus systemic infection or injection with lipopolysaccharide can give rise to uveitis.

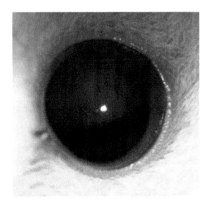

**Figure 7.11**   Hyphaema from hyaloid haemorrhage in a BALB/c mouse.

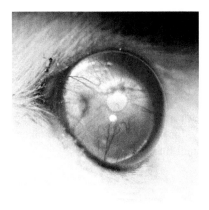

**Figure 7.12**   Buphthalmic globe in a glaucomatous mouse.

### Clinical management

The use of a mydriatic such as atropine and topical anti-inflammatory such as prednisolone acetate or a non-steroidal such as ketorolac will aid in resolving the pathology in uveitis, but identifying and treating the underlying cause is important. Note, however, that the topical use of such agents is likely to give a systemic overdose as nasolacrimal absorption of the majority of the drug will occur in such small eyes.

## Glaucoma

### Clinical signs

In the small globes of the rat and mouse with their thin sclera, any increase in intraocular pressure rapidly leads to an increase in globe size (Figure 7.12). This is the most common sign of glaucoma in these rodent species and, since it occurs rapidly on elevation of intraocular pressure, is more likely to be seen as the first sign of glaucoma than the more subtle signs of episcleral engorgement, mydriasis and visual disturbance which we might expect to see in early glaucoma in the dog or cat.

### Aetiopathogenesis

Glaucoma may be seen in some rats and mice, as inbred strains have been created with a propensity to glaucoma [40–42]. In these animals the mechanism of drainage obstruction is not dysplastic development of the iridocorneal angle, as in the *bu/bu* rabbit or several breeds of dog, but rather the development of peripheral anterior synechiae which occlude the drainage angle in some mice or the deposition of pigment cells in the drainage angle in the DBA mouse model of pigment dispersion. Other rodent models for glaucoma include those in which episcleral vessel occlusion is created by laser photocoagulation [43] or where injection of microspheres into the anterior chamber leads to angle blockade [44]. The optic nerve degeneration seen in glaucoma can be replicated by the optic nerve crush model, but clearly these models in which glaucoma is artificially induced will not be seen in rodents kept as pets.

### Clinical management

Given that many spontaneous cases of glaucoma are related to the development of peripheral anterior synechiae between the iris and cornea, one might hope that anti-inflammatory medication could reduce this. The problem is that once globe enlargement has been noted, the synechial development has occurred and cannot be reversed. Use of drugs to reduce ocular hypertension could be considered, but one problem in these small animals is that the delivery of a substantial dose of carbonic anhydrase inhibitors or adrenergic agonists, as might be used in a dog or cat, can deliver substantial drug doses systemically because of trans-conjunctival and trans-nasolacrimal absorption. Given the risk of this systemic absorption in man with subsequent bronchoconstriction, there is a substantial interest in the degree of systemic absorption in rodent models of topical ocular medications [45].

## Cataract

### Clinical signs

Opacification of the lens is similar across species but the small size of the rodent eye means that most cataracts are not detected, unless by one looking specifically for them with an ophthalmoscope or slit lamp biomicroscope, until they are mature or near mature. At this stage the entire lens, or the majority of it, is an opalescent white (Figures 7.13 and 7.14). Use of a slit lamp biomicroscope, or even a direct ophthalmoscope at +10 D can give a magnified view which improves cataract detection quite substantially. If animals are being used in an experimental setting, especially in a drug-screening protocol, the onset of a lens opacity not caused by the agent in question would be a significant confounding factor in the study. It is therefore important to know whether the animals

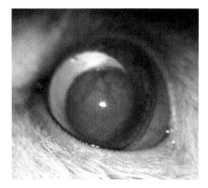

**Figure 7.13**   Nuclear cataract in a rat.

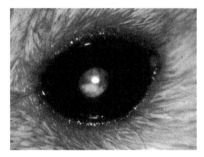

**Figure 7.14**   Immature but progressing cataract in an outbred mouse.

being used have a predisposition to cataract formation through genetic or environmental agencies.

### Aetiopathogenesis

A number of rat and mouse strains have inherited cataract, created or specifically bred from a spontaneous mutation, as a model for human cataract [46,47]. Thus mutations of a number of genes in the lens can be critical in the development of congenital cataracts. Examples include the crystallin protein molecules which make up the bulk of the lens, the ion channels critical in stablising the amount of water in the lens and the enzymes, such as superoxide dismutase, which ensure a correct redox status for the lens and ensure that photo-oxidation of crystallins is minimised.

Indeed even age-related cataracts, which one might expect to be predominantly environmentally mediated, have a genetic component, as shown by Wolf's work on cataractogenesis in older individuals of a number of different strains [48]. Evaluating both cataracts and posterior synechiae in a heterogeneous mouse population obtained by four-way back crossing, three alleles on chromosomes 4, 11 and 12 were determined to be particularly important in the development of these lens opacities [49].

Cataracts can occur secondary to effects from other ocular disease such as retinal degenerations (see below) where lipid peroxidation biproducts are the most likely agency through which cataract is caused [50]. Having said that, cataract is relatively common in RCS rats with a retinal pigment epithelial degeneration [51] but not in mice with the rd mutation of the phosphodiesterase enzyme within the phototransduction cascade [52]. Interestingly cataract in the RCS rat can be delayed by the inclusion of sunflower kernels in the diet [53] and by rearing the animals in the dark [54]. Diabetic mice and rats develop cataracts rapidly and the anti-oxidant pyruvate can delay their onset and reduce their severity [55], as it can in experimentally induced ultraviolet-mediated cataracts [56].

### Clinical management

In most cases rats and mice live an apparently normal life when blinded by lens opacification. The small size of the eye renders cataract extraction difficult and thus the cost–benefit analysis of surgery normally lies on the side of what we might call benign neglect. As might be expected, no reports are extant of cataract surgery in these small rodents from the veterinary literature. Experimental studies of capsular opacification after cataract surgery in the rat have used extracapsular techniques for lens removal but the use of such techniques in the rat or mouse are not generally considered justifiable [57].

## Lens luxation

### Clinical signs

Lens luxation has been reported in rodents but occurs rarely [58]. Generally the lens can be observed in the anterior chamber with an aphakic crescent evident where the lens has slipped ventrally.

### Aetiopathology

Lens luxation in rodents is most commonly secondary to globe enlargement following glaucoma. It has also been noted as an effect of soft X-ray irradiation *in utero* [59].

### Clinical management

The small size of the rat and mouse eye make surgery to remove the lens taxing and ensuing glaucoma is problematic. In most cases, as noted above, the luxation is secondary to globe enlargement and thus lendectomy is not curative anyway.

## Vitreal haemorrhage

### Clinical signs

A substantial number of laboratory rodents have vitreal haemorrhage associated with retained hyaloid vasculature as noted above (Figure 7.11). Some individuals have aneurysms which can rupture giving intravitreal haemorrhage (Figure 7.15).

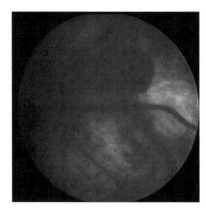

**Figure 7.15**    Saccular aneurysm of retinal vessels in an adult F344 rat. (Reproduced courtesy of Mr Peter Lee.)

### Aetiopathogenesis

It might be asked why so many rodents have retained vasculature with resulting vitreal bleeds. In some studies these changes are seen in older rodents so the lesions may develop over time. The haemorrhages can also be associated with preretinal vascular loops which, with minor trauma, bleed uncontrollably.

### Clinical management

It has to be said that, given the mostly nocturnal habits of these animals and their relatively poor visual acuity, treatment of vitreal haemorrhages is generally not required. If intraocular pressure increases through blood clotting in the iridocorneal angle or aqueous draining vessels, treatment might be necessary to reduce intraocular pressure using topical carbonic anhydrase inhibitors or prostaglandin analogues. The major problem posed by these vitreal haemorrhages is that they preclude visualisation of the retina in many cases, thus hampering experimental studies when the rodents are held in a research environment.

## Retinal degeneration

### Clinical signs

As noted above most rodents are nocturnal or crepuscular animals, active from dusk until dawn. That means that vision is not anything like as important to them as to the companion animal species we are perhaps more used to dealing with. Thus a completely blind mouse may appear completely normal in its behaviour and interactions with other animals, at least to an untrained observer, unless specific tests such as the Morris water maze are used. Clinically, pupil dilation may be evident, although not invariably so. In a laboratory setting specific behavioural tests such as the water maze can give an indication of vision, although even an apparently clear test in other species such as the vertical drop test needs to be interpreted with caution as a simple measure of visual capability in these species.

### Aetiopathogenesis

A significant number of mice used in laboratory research, and indeed available as pet animals, come from stock, such as the C3H strain, affected with the rd gene mutation. This prevents the action of retinal phosphodiesterase, a key player in the phototransduction pathway leading from a photon of light activating rhodopsin. Other strains of mouse and rat especially prone to blindness, are albino animals where retinal damage normally occurs through light damage to the retina, since even if the lids are closed shut, light can still impinge on the retina.

### Clinical management

Most of these animals appear unaffected by their blindness, at least to a human observer. Behavioural assessment has shown that blind animals have increased duration and intensity of aggressive territorial behaviour, perhaps because they cannot visualise the body postures of their adversaries [60]. Having said that, olfactory and auditory cues are so much more important to most of these rodent strains, that defective vision may not be all that important from a welfare perspective. Thus management of these animals once blind is not perhaps that taxing an issue although it should not be overlooked when assessing the welfare of an individual animal or a group.

What might be more important are steps to prevent blindness in the first place. Use of animals not affected by the rd mutation in transgenic and other research would be a valuable first step. Ensuring that animals, and especially albino strains, are not exposed to high levels of illumination, especially on the top row of cages on a stacking system is also very important. Photic damage leading to blindness can occur very quickly and thus all possible steps should be taken to ensure that animals are not over-illuminated. This will include the use of red plastic containers as areas where the animals can rest. These are dark to the rodents, whose retinas have spectral sensitivities highest in the blue wavelengths, as noted above, and also serve to filter out the higher-energy light from the blue end of the spectrum, which causes photic damage to the retina. In the home environment encountered by pet animals this is likely to be less of a problem, but still it is worth warning owners of the hazards of keeping albino animals in a continuously high-light environment.

## Ocular neoplasms

### Clinical signs

Many different rat and mouse strains have been bred with a propensity to develop tumours in various sites from the mammary carcinomas to intracranial neuromas, and the eye is potentially affected by many tumours in these rodent species.

# References

1. Williams DL. Ocular disease in rats: a review. Vet Ophthalmol 2002;5:183–191.
2. Smith RS, John SWM, Nishina PM, Sundberg JP (eds). *Systematic Evaluation of the Mouse Eye; Anatomy, Pathology and Biomethods*. Boca Raton: CRC Press, 2002.
3. Djeridane Y. Comparative histological and ultrastructural studies of the Harderian gland of rodents. Microsc Res Tech 1996;34:28–38.
4. Williams RA, Howard AG, Williams TP. Retinal damage in pigmented and albino rats exposed to low levels of cyclic light following a single mydriatic treatment. Curr Eye Res 1985;4: 97–102.
5. Timm KI. Orbital venous anatomy of the rat. Lab Anim Sci 1979;29:636–638.
6. Timm KI. Orbital venous anatomy of the Mongolian gerbil with comparison to the mouse, hamster and rat. Lab Anim Sci 1989;39:262–264.
7. Guyomard JL, Rosolen SG, Paques M, Delyfer MN, Simonutti M, Tessier Y, Sahel JA, Legargasson JF, Picaud S. A low-cost and simple imaging technique of the anterior and posterior segments: eye fundus, ciliary bodies, iridocorneal angle. Invest Ophthalmol Vis Sci 2008;49:5168–5174.
8. Xiao W, Wu Y, Zhang J, Ye W, Xu GT. Selecting highly sensitive non-obese diabetic mice for improving the study of Sjögren's syndrome. Graefes Arch Clin Exp Ophthalmol 2009;247: 59–66.
9. Morrison JC, Jia L, Cepurna W, Guo Y, Johnson E. Reliability and sensitivity of the TonoLab rebound tonometer in awake Brown Norway rats. Invest Ophthalmol Vis Sci 2009;50: 2802–2808.
10. Szél A, Röhlich P, Caffé AR, Juliusson B, Aguirre G, Van Veen T. Unique topographic separation of two spectral classes of cones in the mouse retina. J Comp Neurol 1992;325:327–342.
11. Jacobs GH, Fenwick JA, Williams GA. Cone-based vision of rats for ultraviolet and visible lights. J Exp Biol 2001;204:2439–2446.
12. Szél A, Röhlich P, Caffé AR, van Veen T Distribution of cone photoreceptors in the mammalian retina. Microsc Res Tech 1996;35:445–462.
13. Prusky GT, Harker KT, Douglas RM, Whishaw IQ. Variation in visual acuity within pigmented, and between pigmented and albino rat strains. Behav Brain Res 2002;136:339–348
14. Birch D, Jacobs GH. Spatial contrast sensitivity in albino and pigmented rats. Vision Res 1979;19:933–937.
15. Curcio CA, Allen KA. Topography of ganglion cells in human retina. J Comp Neurol 1990;300:5–25.
16. Heffner RS, Heffner HE. Visual factors in sound localization in mammals. J Comp Neurol 1992;317:219–232.
17. Hubel DH, Wiesel TN. Receptive fields, binocular interaction and functional architecture in the cat's visual centres. J Physiol 1960;160:106–154.
18. Prusky GT, Reidel C, Douglas RM. Environmental enrichment from birth enhances visual acuity but not place learning in mice. Behav Brain Res 2000;114:11–15.
19. Prusky GT, West PW, Douglas RM. Experience-dependent plasticity of visual acuity in rats. Eur J Neurosci 2000;12:3781–3786.
20. Prusky GT, Douglas RM. Developmental plasticity of mouse visual acuity. Eur J Neurosci 2003;17:167–173.
21. Iny K, Heynen AJ, Sklar E, Bear MF. Bidirectional modifications of visual acuity induced by monocular deprivation in juvenile and adult rats. J Neurosci 2006;26:7368–374.
22. Prusky GT, Alam NM, Douglas RM. Enhancement of vision by monocular deprivation in adult mice. J Neurosci 2006;26:11554–11561.

23. Legg CR, Lambert S. Distance estimation in the hooded rat: experimental evidence for the role of motion cues. Behav Brain Res 1990;41:11–20.

24. Ilia M, Jeffery G. Retinal cell addition and rod production depend on early stages of ocular melanin synthesis. J Comp Neurol 2000;420:437–444.

25. Grant S, Patel NN, Philp AR, Grey CN, Lucas RD, Foster RG, Bowmaker JK, Jeffery G. Rod photopigment deficits in albinos are specific to mammals and arise during retinal development. Vis Neurosci 2001;18:245–251.

26. Muntz WR. A behavioural study on photopic and scotopic vision in the hooded rat. Vision Res 1967;7:371–376.

27. Harkness JE, Ridgway MD. Chromodacryorrhoea in laboratory rats (*Rattus norvegicus*): etiologic considerations. Lab Anim Sci 1980;30:841–844.

28. Kurisu K, Sawamoto O, Watanabe H, Ito A. Sequential changes in the Harderian gland of rats exposed to high intensity light. Lab Anim Sci 1996;46:71–76.

29. Young C, Hill A. Conjunctivitis in a colony of rats. Lab Anim 1974;8:301–304.

30. Innes JRM, Stanton MF. Acute disease of the submaxillary and Harderian glands (sialodacryoadenitis) of rats with cytomegaly and no inclusion bodies. Am J Pathol 1961;38:455–468.

31. Carthew P, Slinger RP. Diagnosis of sialodacryoadenitis virus infection of rats in a virulent enzootic outbreak. Lab Anim 1981;15:339–342.

32. Bhatt PN, Jacoby RO. Epizootological observations of natural and experimental infection with sialodacryoadenitis virus in rats. Lab Anim Sci 1985;35:129–134.

33. Hanna PE, Percy DH, Paturzo F, Bhatt PN. Sialodacryoadenitis in the rat: effects of immunosuppression on the course of the disease. Am J Vet Res 1984;45:2077–2083.

34. Gannon J, Carthew P. Prevalence of indigenous viruses in laboratory animal colonies in the United Kingdom 1978–79. Lab Anim 1980;14:309–311.

35. Kinney HC, Klintworth GK, Lesiewicz J, Goldsmith LA, Wilkening B. Congenital cystic microphthalmia and consequent anophthalmia in the rat: a study in abnormal ocular morphogenesis. Teratology 1982;26(2):203–212.

36. Smith RS, Roderick TH, Sundberg JP. Microphthalmia and associated abnormalities in inbred black mice. Lab Anim Sci 1994;44(6):551–560.

37. Robinson ML, Holmgren A, Dewey MJ. Genetic control of ocular morphogenesis: defective lens development associated with ocular anomalies in C57BL/6 mice. Exp Eye Res 1993; 56:7–16.

38. Park SA, Jeong SM, Yi NY, Kim MS, Jeong MB, Suh JG, Oh YS, Won MH, Nam TC, Park JH, Seo KM. Study on the ophthalmic diseases in ICR mice and BALB/c mice. Exp Anim 2006;55:83–90.

39. Heywood R. Some clinical observations on the eyes of Sprague-Dawley rats. Lab Anim 1973; 7:19–27.

40. Sheldon WG, Warbritton AR, Bucci TJ, Turturro A Glaucoma in food-restricted and ad libitum-fed DBA/2NNia mice. Lab Anim Sci 1995;45:508–518.

41. John SW, Smith RS, Savinova OV, Hawes NL, Chang B, Turnbull D, Davisson M, Roderick TH, Heckenlively JR. Essential iris atrophy, pigment dispersion, and glaucoma in DBA/2J mice. Invest Ophthalmol Vis Sci 1998;39:951–962.

42. McKinnon SJ, Schlamp CL, Nickells RW. Mouse models of retinal ganglion cell death and glaucoma. Exp Eye Res 2009;88:816–824.

43. Aihara M, Lindsey JD, Weinreb RN. Experimental mouse ocular hypertension: establishment of the model. Invest Ophthalmol Vis Sci 2003;44:4314–4320.

44. Urcola JH, Hernández M, Vecino E. Three experimental glaucoma models in rats: comparison of the effects of intraocular pressure elevation on retinal ganglion cell size and death. Exp Eye Res 2006;83:429–437.

45. Tan AY, LeVatte TL, Archibald ML, Tremblay F, Kelly ME, Chauhan BC. Timolol concentrations in rat ocular tissues and plasma after topical and intraperitoneal dosing. J Glaucoma 2002;11:134–142.

46. Graw J. Mouse models of congenital cataract. Eye (Lond) 1999;13:438–444.

47. Tripathi BJ, Tripathi RC, Borisuth NS, Dhaliwal R, Dhaliwal D. Rodent models of congenital and hereditary cataract in man. Lens Eye Toxic Res 1991;8:373–413.

48. Wolf N, Penn P, Pendergrass W, Van Remmen H, Bartke A, Rabinovitch P, Martin GM. Age-related cataract progression in five mouse models for anti-oxidant protection or hormonal influence. Exp Eye Res 2005;81:276–285.

49. Wolf N, Galecki A, Lipman R, Chen S, Smith-Wheelock M, Burke D, Miller R. Quantitative trait locus mapping for age-related cataract severity and synechia prevalence using four-way cross mice. Invest Ophthalmol Vis Sci 2004;45:1922–1929.

50. Zigler JS Jr, Hess HH. Cataracts in the Royal College of Surgeons rat: evidence for initiation by lipid peroxidation products. Exp Eye Res 1985;41:67–76.

51. Al-ghoul KJ, Novak LA, Kuszak JR. The structure of posterior subcapsular cataracts in the Royal College of Surgeons (RCS) rats. Exp Eye Res 1998;67:163–177.

52. Carper D, Russell P, Sanyal S. Comparison of the lens crystallin proteins from normal, rd, and rds mutant mice utilizing specific monoclonal antibodies. Exp Eye Res 1985;40:757–761.

53. Hess HH, Knapka JJ, Newsome DA, Westney IV, Wartofsky L. Dietary prevention of cataracts in the pink-eyed RCS rat. Lab Anim Sci 1985;35:47–53.

54. O'Keefe TL, Hess HH, Zigler JS Jr, Kuwabara T, Knapka JJ. Prevention of cataracts in pink-eyed RCS rats by dark rearing. Exp Eye Res 1990;51:509–517.

55. Varma SD, Hegde KR, Kovtun S. Attenuation and delay of diabetic cataracts by antioxidants: effectiveness of pyruvate after onset of cataract. Ophthalmologica 2005;219:309–315.

56. Hegde KR, Kovtun S, Varma SD. Induction of ultraviolet cataracts in vitro: prevention by pyruvate. J Ocul Pharmacol Ther 2007;23:492–502.

57. Lois N, Dawson R, McKinnon A, Forrester JV. A new model of posterior capsule opacification in rodents. Invest Ophthalmol Vis Sci 2003;44:3450–3457.

58. Takizawa Y, Sakasai K, Harada T, Ebino KY. Lens luxation in a CD-1 mouse. Exp Anim 1996;45:271–273.

59. Kuno H, Kemi M, Akimoto M, Fujii T, Usui T. Effects of soft X-ray irradiation on ocular development in Sprague-Dawley rats. Jikken Dobutsu 1993;42:443–449.

60. Strasser S, Dixon AK. Effects of visual and acoustic deprivation on agonistic behaviour of the albino mouse (*M. musculus L.*). Physiol Behav 1986;36:773–778.

# Chapter 8

# The eye of other mammalian exotic pet species

## Introduction

Apart from the rat and mouse, the rabbit and guinea pig, a number of other mammalian species are regularly kept as pets. The smaller rodents, such as hamsters and gerbils, and larger species, including chinchillas and degus, have specific ocular problems but there is insufficient data on these to warrant whole chapters for each species. Primates might be considered rather a different case in point. They are infrequently kept as companion animals but clearly do have ophthalmic problems worthy of inclusion. Thus in this chapter we will consider specific problems for each species group but in less detail than in previous chapters.

## Hamsters

While many hamsters are kept in laboratory colonies, the only literature on eye diseases in the species are individual case reports from anophthalmos in a colour dilute strain [1], through multifocal retinal dysplasia [2] to metastatic eyelid melanomas [3] and suspected keratoconjunctivitis sicca [4], although anecdotal evidence would suggest a higher prevalence of the latter condition than the single case in the literature suggests. The problem with this last condition is that the hamster palpebral aperture is too small for a Schirmer tear test. The phenol red thread test (PRTT) can be a useful alternative in these small eyes but no normal values are available for PRTT readings in this or any other small rodent species. In such cases measurement of tear production in a normal cage-mate or in the normal fellow eye in unilateral cases is valuable. Conjunctivitis can be seen in hamsters, as with all small rodents, where dusty bedding is provided, and the finding of ocular irritation warrants evaluation of the animals' environment quite as much as clinical examination of their eyes.

A common problem with hamsters is globe prolapse either through trauma or from over-enthusiastic handling and 'scruffing' the animal. Normally globes can be readily repositioned but prolonged globe prolapse will lead to exposure keratitis and ocular surface damage. In such cases a tarsoraphy may be appropriate until orbital inflammation

*Ophthalmology of Exotic Pets*, First Edition. David L. Williams.
© 2012 David Williams. Published 2012 by Blackwell Publishing Ltd.

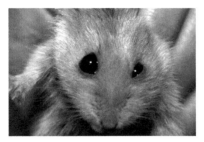

**Figure 8.1**   Buphthalmic globe in a hamster with uveitis and glaucoma.

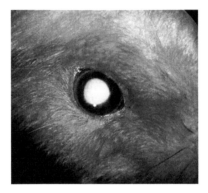

**Figure 8.2**   Mature cataract in an aged hamster.

is reduced. Proptosis can also be seen with globe enlargement – the thin sclera of many small rodent globes predisposes them to globe enlargement with even small increases in intraocular pressure (Figure 8.1).

The Harderian gland of Syrian hamsters (*Mesocricetus auratus*) is unusual in that it exhibits marked sexual dismorphism with the gland of the female having only one cell type secreting small lipid droplets while the males have two types, the second producing much larger lipid drops [5]. Siberian (Djungarian) hamsters (*Phodopus sungorus*) do not exhibit this sexual dimorphism. Male glands of *Mesocricetus* produce significantly less porphyrin than does the female gland although phenotype is also dependent on photoperiod [6] and daylength. The exact function of the gland and its secretions is unclear compared to research on that of the gerbil (see below) where Harderian gland secretions can also be a clinical problem, not generally seen in the hamster.

Cataracts are relatively common in hamsters (Figure 8.2) either solely in older animals or as part of a systemic syndrome such as that seen in cardiomyopathic strains [7].

## Gerbils

The Harderian glands of gerbils produce a copious secretion which can cause facial dermatitis in extreme cases [8]. Removal of the gland alleviates the dermatitis [9] but

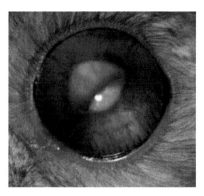

**Figure 8.3**   Lens luxation in a chinchilla.

this should be a last resort given the importance of glandular secretions in several physiological and behavioural functions. The Harderian exudates are central in communication between sexually active gerbils [10]; since they are spread through the hair coat during grooming, they also play a part in thermoregulation [11] and osmotic balance [12].

While the gerbil is an important model for ocular toxacariasis [13] with findings of exudative and haemorrhagic chorioretinitis and vitritis; the parasite does not seem to affect animals in the wild or those kept as pets.

## Chinchillas

A report of ocular findings in a laboratory colony of chinchillas found few major ophthalmic problems, with posterior cortical cataracts and asteroid hyalosis in two animals [14]. Lens luxation has also been noted in chinchillas (Figure 8.3) and this may be managed surgically, although the eye is too small to allow extraction by phacoemulsification. Any ensuing rise in intraocular pressure can be managed with topical ocular antihypertensives such as doszolamide (Trusopt). Dental disease is quite widely seen in these animals in captivity [15], possibly related to calcium deficiency as has been shown in the rabbit with similarly hypsodont (continually growing) teeth. These dental changes often result in epiphora, and dental investigation in such animals, even including diagnostic imaging techniques such as computerised tomography [16], is valuable if the ocular problems are to be controlled. While one might expect cases of exophthalmos in this species to be similarly related to dental disease, one case report shows that other factors, such as a parasitic cyst, have to be taken into consideration [17].

## Degus

The degu, a rodent native to Chile [18], is a species the excellence of whose eyesight has been demonstrated by tool use and manipulation of tiny seeds [19]. Its main interest from an ophthalmic perspective, though, is its propensity to diabetes and the rapidity

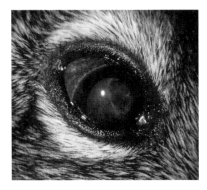

**Figure 8.4** Diabetic cataract in a degu.

with which it develops diabetic cataract (Figure 8.4); this is probably related to the high level of aldose reductase in its lens. This enzyme system, which catalyses the metabolism of glucose into insoluble sugars such as sorbitol, is important in the generation of cataract in diabetic lenses, as shown by the ability of aldose reductase inhibition to prevent cataract formation in the degu lens [20].

# Hedgehogs

The small size of the eye of the European hedgehog (*Erinaceus europaeus*) or the African pygmy hedgehog (*Atelerix albiventris*), more commonly kept as a pet animal, means that many ocular problems probably go unnoticed. Conditions that cause obvious changes to the appearance of the eye or that manifest as ocular pain are more likely to be recognised by those keeping these animals. Thus in the literature the only ophthalmic condition reported in these animals is that of exophthalmos or globe proptosis [21–23]. The shallow orbit of these species also contributes to the high incidence of globe protrusion – 15% of the hedgehogs examined in one veterinary college had exophthalmos as their presenting complaint either with orbital inflammation or neoplasia [21].

Our specific study of ocular disease in hedgehogs is still in its infancy but preliminary results show that many apparently normal-sighted hedgehogs have considerable proptosis and strabismus (Figure 8.5). The close proximity of the spines to the ocular surface and the tendency of hedgehogs to roll into a ball renders trichiasis a common occurrence (Figure 8.6). This normally results in excess tear production and overflow with mucoid conjunctivitis (Figure 8.7) but may give rise to traumatic injury to the eye. Thus the finding of apparent anophthalmos or clinical microphthalmos in some hedgehogs (Figure 8.8) may be cases of phthysis bulbi after chronic injury rather than a congenital defect – we have considerably more work to do in this area to determine the exact aetiopathogenesis of the condition. Other damage to the hedgehog eye can result from fly strike where eggs have been laid around the eyes, with the maggots hatching from these literally eating the eyes away.

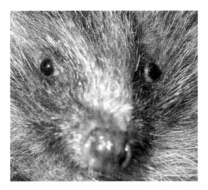

**Figure 8.5**  Apparent exophthalmos in a normal hedgehog.

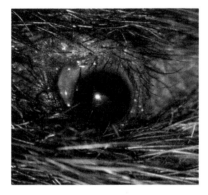

**Figure 8.6**  Entropion with trichiasis in a 3-month-old hedgehog.

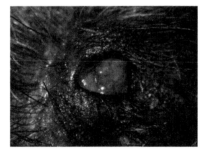

**Figure 8.7**  Anophthalmos in a neonatal hedgehog.

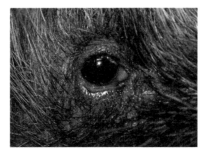

**Figure 8.8**  Epiphora and conjunctivitis in a 3-month-old hedgehog.

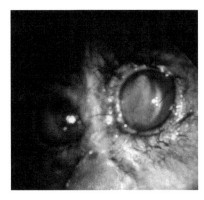

**Figure 8.9**  Keratoconjunctivitis with corneal ulceration in a slender loris.

# Primates

Non-human primates sit in an unusual position, given that on the one hand in many ways ophthalmic diagnostics and therapeutics can be extrapolated from more conventional companion animal species but that on the other their eyes more closely resemble those of humans. Examination should be undertaken under sedation and restraint in the vast majority of cases. The assistance of a medical ophthalmologist may be beneficial given the similarity between non-human primate and human eyes [24]. The literature about ocular disease in these animals is mostly in the form of case reports as will be seen below, but hopefully a review of these will aid those needing to treat similar cases and, indeed, novel ocular lesions in these animals.

Young monkeys are often somewhat esotropic or cross-eyed and in the majority of cases this resolves over the first few weeks of life [25], although some remain with strabismus for much longer and may form a useful model for human strabismus [26]. Congenital anomalies have been reported in primates [27] but are rarely amenable to correction.

Conjunctivitis in primate colonies can be infectious with viral agents as a cause [28]; while parasitic [29], sterile [30] and allergic conjunctivitis have also been reported [31]. Conjunctivitis may be a presenting sign of systemic disease such as coccidiomycosis and clearly a full clinical examination is required in such cases [32].

Other causes of conjunctival hyperaemia include keratoconjunctivitis sicca which, as with dogs and humans, can be treated with topical cyclosporine [33]. Reference values for measurements such as Schirmer tear tests have been published for the capuchin monkey (*Cebus apella*) [34] but will be different for each primate species – comparison with readings from the normal fellow eye or in cases of bilateral disease of a cage-mate of the same species is suggested where values are unknown. This was the case with two slender lorises (*Loris tardigradus*) diagnosed with dry eye when presented with central corneal ulcers and mild changes in their behaviour (Figure 8.9). While twice daily topical cyclosporine medication was effective in increasing tear production, the regular handling required was detrimental to their wellbeing and it was decided that keeping them without treatment was better than giving regular lacrimomimetic medication.

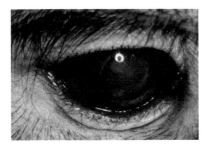

**Figure 8.10**   Cataract in an aged cynomolgus macaque.

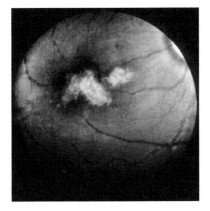

**Figure 8.11**   Focal postinflammatory macular degeneration in a macaque.

Entropion with resultant keratitis has been noted in a macaque and successfully treated with just the same surgery as would be used in a dog [35]. Here extrapolation from the known to the unknown is quite justified. On the other hand some diseases are unique to primates; adnexal changes of molluscum contagiosum have been reported in chimpanzees with these warty swellings otherwise only noted in humans [36]. While such cases are rare, a survey of ocular disease in marmosets and tamarins found almost 10% to have meibomian gland obstructions present with yellow–white waxy material at the meibomian gland orifice and eyelid swelling in some animals [37].

Glaucoma is seen in laboratory primates as an experimentally induced condition but also as a spontaneous disease in a number of cases. The similarity of the aqueous drainage system in primates to that in humans renders such spontaneous disease highly interesting but also of relevance to individual monkeys kept as companion animals. Glaucoma in vervet monkeys has been reported [38] as has raised intraocular pressure in a number of macaques in a large colony derived from an island off the coast of Puerto Rico and maintained in a colony in Gainesville, Florida, since 1930 [39,40]. Glaucoma has also been reported in prosimians with the disease noted in lemurs [41].

Cataracts are relatively common in captive non-human primates (Figure 8.10) and phacofragmentation has been reported in a number of individual animals [42]. Two young related lowland gorillas were diagnosed with cataract and had surgery with intraocular

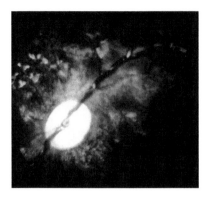

**Figure 8.12**   Retinitis, vasculitis and cotton wool spots in a macaque.

lens implantation [43]. Posterior capsular opacification led to secondary cataract which required Neodynium Yag laser treatment to restore vision. Interestingly lens opacification has been reported in wild-caught African green monkeys with inheritance determined in two reports of cataract in this species [44].

Fundus lesions are also relatively common. A survey of more than 2000 cynomolgus macaques showed a 6.6% prevalence of pathological change, mostly involving chorioretinal scarring which was chronic in nature (Figure 8.11). Some of the fundus lesions were active with vasculitis, retinal haemorrhage and so-called cotton-wool spots indicative of retinal inflammation and oedema (Figure 8.12) [45,46].

The Floridean primate colony noted above has also yielded an important study on ageing change in the primate fundus, specifically regarding drusen and macular degeneration [47,48]. Such changes may also be encountered in older primates kept as companion animals but as they have little influence on vision and there is no treatment their relevance might be said to be primarily academic [49].

## References

1. Asher JH Jr, James SC. The primary ultrastructural defect caused by anophthalmic white (Wh) in the Syrian hamster. Proc Natl Acad Sci U S A 1982;79:4371–4375.
2. Schiavo DM. Multifocal retinal dysplasia in the Syrian hamster LAK:LVG (SYR). J Environ Pathol Toxicol 1980;3:569–576.
3. Mangkoewidjojo S, Kim JC. Malignant melanoma metastatic to the lung in a pet hamster. Lab Anim 1977;11:125–127.
4. Atkinson M. Suspected keratitis sicca in a Syrian hamster. Vet Rec 2000;146:680.
5. Buzzell GR, Blank JL, Vaughan MK, Reiter RJ. Control of secretory lipid droplets in the harderian gland by testosterone and the photoperiod: comparison of two species of hamsters. Gen Comp Endocrinol 1995;99:230–238.
6. Coto-Montes AM, Rodríguez-Colunga MJ, Uría H, Antolin I, Tolivia D, Buzzell GR, Menéndez-Peláez A. Photoperiod and the pineal gland regulate the male phenotype of the Harderian glands of male Syrian hamsters after androgen withdrawal. J Pineal Res 1994;17: 48–54.

7. Thakar JH, Percy DH, Strickland KP. Ocular abnormalities in the myopathic hamster (UM-X7.1 strain). Invest Ophthalmol Vis Sci 1977;16:1047–1052.

8. Thiessen DD, Pendergrass M. Harderian gland involvement in facial lesions in the Mongolian gerbil. J Am Vet Med Assoc 1982;181:1375–1377.

9. Farrar PL, Opsomer MJ, Kocen JA, Wagner JE. Experimental nasal dermatitis in the Mongolian gerbil: effect of bilateral harderian gland adenectomy on development of facial lesions. Lab Anim Sci 1988;38:72–76.

10. Payne AP. The harderian gland: a tercentennial review. J Anat 1994;185:1–49.

11. Thiessen DD, Harriman AE. Harderian gland exudates in the male *Meriones unguiculatus* regulate female proceptive behavior, aggression, and investigation. J Comp Psychol 1986; 100:85–87.

12. Harriman AE, Thiessen D. Removal of Harderian exudates by sandbathing contributes to osmotic balance in Mongolian gerbils. Physiol Behav 1983;31:317–323.

13. Takayanagi TH, Akao N, Suzuki R, Tomoda M, Tsukidate S, Fujita K. New animal model for human ocular toxocariasis: ophthalmoscopic observation. Br J Ophthalmol 1999;83: 967–972.

14. Peiffer RL, Johnson PT. Clinical ocular findings in a colony of chinchillas (*Chinchilla laniger*). Lab Anim 1980;14:331–335.

15. Crossley DA. Dental disease in chinchillas in the UK. J Small Anim Pract 2001;42:12–19.

16. Crossley DA, Jackson A, Yates J, Boydell IP. Use of computed tomography to investigate cheek tooth abnormalities in chinchillas (*Chinchilla laniger*). J Small Anim Pract 1998;39: 385–389.

17. Holmberg BJ, Hollingsworth SR, Osofsky A, Tell LA. Taenia coenurus in the orbit of a chinchilla. Vet Ophthalmol 2007;10:53–59.

18. Lee TM. *Octodon degus*: a diurnal, social, and long-lived rodent. ILAR J 2004; 45:14–24.

19. Okanoya K, Tokimoto N, Kumazawa N, Hihara S, Iriki A. Tool-use training in a species of rodent: the emergence of an optimal motor strategy and functional understanding. PLoS One 2008;3:e1860.

20. Datiles MB 3rd, Fukui H. Cataract prevention in diabetic *Octodon degus* with Pfizer's sorbinil. Curr Eye Res 1989;8:233–237.

21. Wheler CL, Grahn BH, Pocknell AM. Unilateral proptosis and orbital cellulitis in eight African hedgehogs (*Atelerix albiventris*). J Zoo Wildl Med 2001;32:236–241.

22. Fukuzawa R, Fukuzawa K, Abe H, Nagai T, Kameyama K. Acinic cell carcinoma in an African pygmy hedgehog (*Atelerix albiventris*). Vet Clin Pathol 2004;33:39–42.

23. Kuonen VJ, Wilkie DA, Morreale RJ, Oglesbee B, Barrett-Rephun K. Unilateral exophthalmia in a European hedgehog (*Erinaceus europaeus*) caused by a lacrimal ductal carcinoma. Vet Ophthalmol 2002;5:161–165.

24. Liang D, Alvarado TP, Oral D, Vargas JM, Denena MM, McCulley JP. Ophthalmic examination of the captive western lowland gorilla (*Gorilla gorilla gorilla*). J Zoo Wildl Med 2005;36: 430–433.

25. Kiorpes L, Boothe RG. Naturally occurring strabismus in monkeys (*Macaca nemestrina*). Invest Ophthalmol Vis Sci 1981;20:257–263.

26. Narasimhan A, Tychsen L, Poukens V, Demer JL. Horizontal rectus muscle anatomy in naturally and artificially strabismic monkeys. Invest Ophthalmol Vis Sci 2007;48:2576–2588.

27. Ribka EP, Dubielzig RR. Multiple ophthalmic abnormalities in an infant rhesus macaque (*Macaca mulatta*). J Med Primatol 2008;37:16–19.

28. Tyrrell DA, Buckland FE, Lancaster MC, Valentine RC. Some properties of a strain of SV-17 virus isolated from an epidemic of conjunctivitis and rhinorrhoea in monkeys (*Erythrocebus pates*). Br J Exp Pathol 1960;41:610–616.

29. Ivanova E, Spiridonov S, Bain O. Ocular oxyspirurosis of primates in zoos: intermediate host, worm morphology, and probable origin of the infection in the Moscow zoo. Parasite 2007;14: 287–298.

30. Schmidt RE. Ophthalmic lesions in non-human primates. Vet Pathol 1971;8:28–36.

31. Hoopes J, Montali RJ, Ensley PK, Bush M, Koch SA. Allergic conjunctivitis in a juvenile black spider monkey. J Am Vet Med Assoc 1977;171:870–871.

32. Hoffman K, Videan EN, Fritz J, Murphy J. Diagnosis and treatment of ocular coccidioidomycosis in a female captive chimpanzee (*Pan troglodytes*): a case study. Ann N Y Acad Sci 2007; 1111:404–410.

33. Schuler AM, Tustin GT, Abee CR, Scammell JG. Restasis for the treatment of 'dry eye' in *Aotus nancymaae*. J Med Primatol 2009;38:318–320.

34. Montiani-Ferreira F, Shaw G, Mattos BC, Russ HH, Vilani RG. Reference values for selected ophthalmic diagnostic tests of the capuchin monkey (*Cebus apella*). Vet Ophthalmol 2008;11: 197–201.

35. Peiffer RL, Johnson PT, Wilkerson BJ. Peripalpebral folds and entropion in a male crab-eating macaque (*Macaca fasicularis*). Lab Anim Sci 1980;30:113–115.

36. Douglas JD, Tanner KN, Prine JR, Van Riper DC, Derwelis SK. Molluscum contagiosum in chimpanzees. J Am Vet Med Asoc 1967;151:901–904.

37. Buyukimichi N, Richter CB. Prevalence of ocular disease in a colony of tamarins and marmosets. Lab Anim Sci 1979;29:800–804.

38. Barany EH, Rohen JW. Glaucoma in owl monkeys (*Cercopythicus aethiops*). Arch Ophthalmol 1963;69:630.

39. Dawson WW, Brooks DE, Hope GM, Samuelson DA, Sherwood MB, Engel HM, Kessler MJ. Primary open angle glaucomas in the rhesus monkey. Br J Ophthalmol 1993;77:302–310.

40. Dawson WW, Brooks DE, Dawson JC, Sherwood MB, Kessler MJ, Garcia A. Signs of glaucoma in rhesus monkeys from a restricted gene pool. J Glaucoma 1998;7:343–348.

41. Shields MB, Ritch R. Spontaneous buphthalmos in *Lemur fulvus rufus*. Prog Vet Comp Ophthalmol 1991;1:87–91.

42. Whiteley RD, Jacobson ER, Lavach JD, Gelatt KN, Barrie KP. Bilateral ultrasonic phacofragmentation and aspiration cataract extraction in a Spider monkey. J Zool Anim Med 1980;11: 58–60.

43. de Faber JT, Pameijer JH, Schaftenaar W . Cataract surgery with foldable intraocular lens implants in captive lowland gorillas (*Gorilla gorilla gorilla*). J Zoo Wildl Med 2004;35: 520–524.

44. Suzaki MT, Hiyaoka A, Cho F, Fukui M. Some cases of cataract in African green monkeys. Anim Eye Res 1988;7:27–29.

45. Suzuki MT, Cho F: Normal and abnormal findings in ocular fundi of cynomolgus monkeys. J Toxicol Sci 1986;11:452–457.

46. Kuhlman SM, Rubin LF, Ridgeway RL. Prevalence of ophthalmic lesions in wild-caught cynomolgus monkeys. Prog Vet Comp Ophthalmol 1992;2:20–28.

47. Dawson WW, Ulshafer RJ, Engel HM, Hope GM, Kessler MJ. Macular disease in related rhesus monkeys. Doc Ophthalmol. 1989;71:253–263.

48. Suzuki MT, Cho F. Normal and abnormal findings in ocular fundi of cynomolgus monkeys. J Toxicol Sci 1986;11:452–457.

49. Suzuki MT, Ogawa H, Cho F, Honjo S. Visual function in cynomolgus monkeys with macular degeneration. Anim Eye Res 1989;8:33–38.

# Chapter 9

# The avian eye

## Introduction

Vision is centrally important to the vast majority of birds. A fish or lizard can cope with relatively poor resolution to see its prey, a cow does not need to differentiate food items of different colour and a mouse, active for the most part by night, hardly needs sight at all! But a bird in flight landing on a branch, catching insects on the wing, seeking out a prey rodent species on the ground as it hovers above or swooping in a dense flock in the early evening air needs exceptional sight. It was this very realisation that made the Canadian ophthalmologist Casey Albert Wood, whom we met in Chapter 2, study birds and their vision so intensely in the later part of the nineteenth and the early years of the twentieth century. His aim was to find ways of improving human visual capabilities by investigating quite what made avian vision so good. For veterinarians this feature of the avian sensory world means that maintaining optimal vision in the birds under our care should be a priority.

## Anatomy and physiology of the avian eye

If we say that vision is vitally important to birds then understanding the anatomy and physiology of the avian eye and how it differs from that of other species is crucial in arriving at a correct diagnosis of avian ocular disease and critical in differentiating the abnormal from the considerable range of normal variations. The key monograph in avian ophthalmic basic sciences is that of Professor Graham Martin [1], of whom more later. A more concise coverage can be found from Willis and Wilkie who have reviewed the subject area in two relatively recent papers [2].

We should consider first the avian eyelids. Both are mobile but the lower considerably more so than the upper. The Meibomian glands are absent but the lacrimal gland is present inferior and lateral to the globe with an additional Harderian gland acting as a second lacrimal gland at the base of the nictitating membrane. The nictitating membrane moves over the cornea during blinking and the menace response, drawn across by an unusual muscle arrangement. The pyramidalis muscle, which accomplishes this action,

*Ophthalmology of Exotic Pets*, First Edition. David L. Williams.
© 2012 David Williams. Published 2012 by Blackwell Publishing Ltd.

originates on the posterior sclera and loops around the optic nerve through a sling formed by the bursalis muscle, also known as the quadratus muscle (Figure 9.1). Inferior and superior nasolacrimal puncta drain the lacrimal secretions into the nasal cavity.

The orbit is open and is occupied predominantly by the globe in most birds (Figure 9.2). For this reason the extraocular muscles are not particularly well developed in those

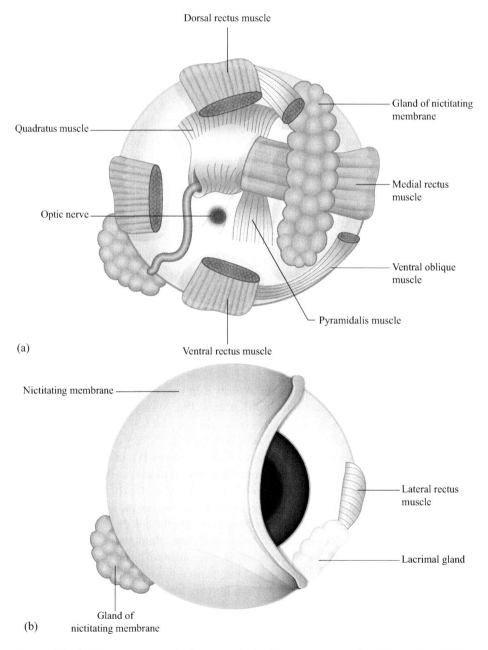

**Figure 9.1**   (a) The arrangement of muscles behind the eye moving the third eyelid. (b) The nictitating membrane extended over the ocular surface.

species. Torsional movements of the globe are generally limited to between 2 and 5 degrees. As will be seen later though, such movements are very important to retinal nutrition. The most important feature of the orbit is the close proximity of the globe to the infraorbital diverticulum of the infraorbital sinus (Figure 9.3). Enlargement of this diverticulum in sinusitis leads to a number of conditions from periorbital swelling, orbital compression, conjunctivitis and sometimes exophthalmos or intraocular inflammation. It

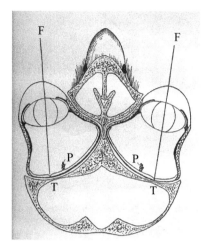

**Figure 9.2**  The orbit almost completely filled by the globe which takes up a substantial proportion of the cranial volume, here shown in a drawing from Casey Wood's 1917 *Fundus Oculi of Birds*.

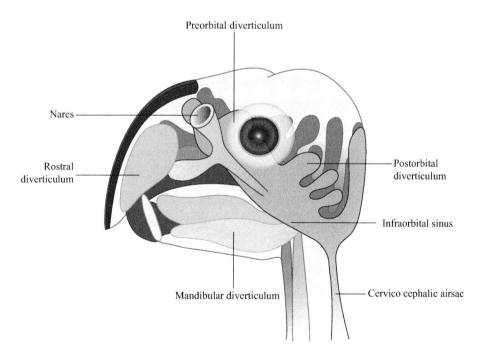

**Figure 9.3**  The sinuses around the eye.

is important to be aware of the extensive network of sinuses in the cranial area in order to appreciate the extent that inflammatory involvement of the sinus system may take.

Different bird species have quite variable globe shape. The majority of birds, including passerines and psittaciformes, have a somewhat anterior–posteriorly flattened globe forming an oblate spheroid with a hemispherical posterior segment (Figure 9.4). In several species of owl, however, the posterior segment is tubular allowing a considerably magnified image to be projected on the retina (Figure 9.5).

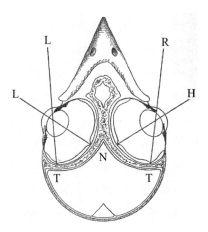

**Figure 9.4**   The ovoid globe of the passerines, from Casey Wood's 1917 *Fundus Oculi of Birds.*

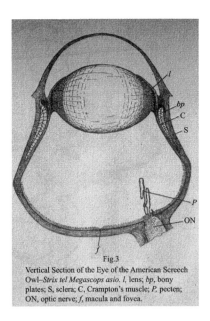

Fig.3
Vertical Section of the Eye of the American Screech
Owl–*Strix tel Megascops asio. l,* lens; *bp,* bony
plates; S, sclera; C, Crampton's muscle; *P,* pecten;
ON, optic nerve; *f,* macula and fovea.

**Figure 9.5**   The tubular globe of the American screech owl, from Casey Wood's 1917 *Fundus Oculi of Birds.*

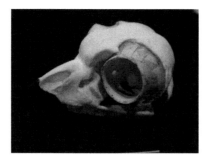

**Figure 9.6**  The ring of scleral ossicles in the owl eye.

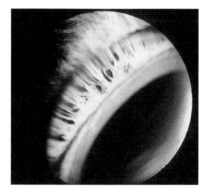

**Figure 9.7**  The iridocorneal angle of an eagle owl.

The avian cornea is similar to that of mammals but for its considerably reduced thickness, an important factor to note when performing corneal surgery, and the fact that its anterior stroma is quite obviously acellular with a marked Bowman's layer, unlike that of subprimate mammals. A more important difference from the mammalian eye is the presence of a ring of scleral ossicles immediately behind the limbus (Figure 9.6). These bony structures are probably important from an anatomical and physiological perspective in providing a firm origin for the muscles which allow accommodation. From a therapeutic perspective they change the approach to enucleation in many birds where they render the surgical removal of the globe more challenging.

The anterior chamber of most avian eyes is considerably shallower than that of mammals, that is with the exception of owls which have a deep anterior chamber. Such differences have clinical implications with regard to examination of the iridocorneal angle which, while taxing in many species, is relatively easy in owls where a goniolens is not required (Figure 9.7).

The avian iris is thin and, importantly, contains striated muscle rather than the autonomically innervated dilator and constrictor muscles of the mammalian eye. This has considerable implications for pharmacological dilation of the pupil, requiring depolarising or, more commonly these days, non-depolarising muscle relaxants rather than the simple and effective parasympatholytic drugs tropicamide or atropine commonly used to produce mydriasis in mammals. This difference in iridal innervation allows birds to consciously control pupil dilation and constriction which can make the iris an important device in communication. For that reason the avian iris can be brightly coloured to allow flashes of iridal constriction to become danger signals or signs of sexual attractiveness. Chromatophores within the avian iris render the iris a sign of sexual dimorphism in some species with the male cockatoo iris being dark brown while the female has a pinkish-red iris. Changes in iris colour can also occur with age; young blue and gold macaws have dark irides which turn yellow as they reach sexual maturity while young African grey parrots have muddy-grey irides which turn a more yellow hue as the bird ages.

The conscious control of pupillary musculature complicates evaluation of the pupillary light reflex. Miosis does occur with retinal stimulation but clearly can also occur in its absence. Another important difference between the avian and mammalian visual system is the absence in the former of decussation at the optic chiasm. Integration of the sensory information from each visual field occurs in the midbrain and this renders the concept of the direct and consensual pupillary light reflex redundant.

The lens of birds differs quite considerably from that of their mammalian counterparts. The lens is generally soft with a conspicuous annular pad lying under the lens capsule in the equatorial region allowing considerable attachment between the lens and the muscles of accommodation.

Accommodation, that is to say change in the focal length of the lens, in the bird is produced by the ciliary muscles which are divided in two portions [3]. The anterior of these is termed Crampton's muscle (Figure 9.8). It originates on the sclera beneath the scleral ossicles and its contraction has the effect of flattening the cornea at its peripheral margin and giving a central bulging effect to the cornea, increasing its refractive power. This gives about 40% of total accommodative power in birds such as the chicken but

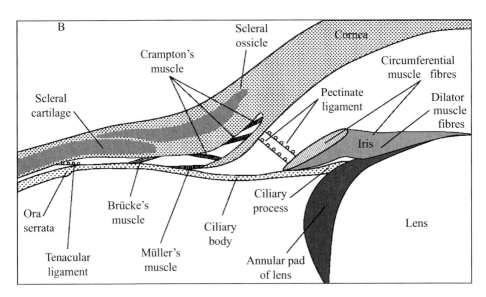

**Figure 9.8** Musculature of accommodation in the bird. Reprinted from *The Quarterly Review of Biology*, Vol. 71, no. 4, Adrian Glasser and Howard C Howland, 'A History of Studies of Visual Accommodation in the Bird' © 1996 University of Chicago Press.

less in raptors where the change is between 2.5 and 6.2 D in a total range of accommodation of 25 D. The posterior component of the ciliary body is the so-called Brucke's muscle which pulls the ciliary body forward, lessening tension applied to the annular pad by the tenacular ligament from the ciliary body. The deformation of the lens is also caused by pressure from the circumferential muscle of the iris which bulges the central portion of the lens into the pupil increasing its refractive power. The density of this circumferential muscle differs between species and is particularly marked in diving birds where the substantial increase in refractive power of the lens makes up for the lack of refractive power of the cornea under water [4].

The retina of the bird differs markedly from that of the mammal. Without retinal blood vessels or a choriocapillaris to provide a direct vascular supply of oxygen and nutrition for the retinal photoreceptors, a portion of the choroid, the pecten, protrudes into the fluid posterior vitreous (Figures 9.9 and 9.10). Continual small torsional movements of the globe cause the pecten to move backwards and forwards in this fluid vitreous with

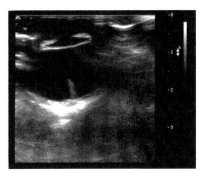

**Figure 9.9**   The pecten, protruding into the posterior vitreous as seen on ultrasonography

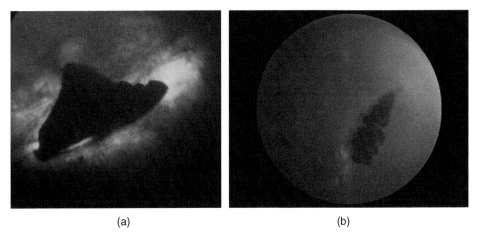

(a)                                                                     (b)

**Figure 9.10**   (a) The pecten and choroidal vasculature of the avian fundus by direct ophthalmoscopy. (b) The pecten and choroidal vasculature of the avian fundus by indirect ophthalmoscopy.

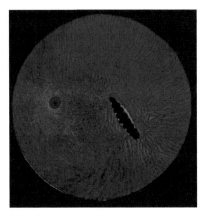

**Figure 9.11**   The distinct fovea of the tawny owl, from Wood's 1917 *Fundus Oculi of Birds.*

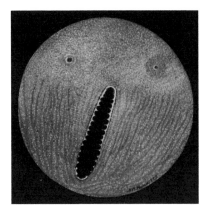

**Figure 9.12**   The two foveolae of the kestrel, from Wood's 1917 *Fundus Oculi of Birds.*

diffusion of both oxygen and nutrients from the vascular elements of the pecten across the posterior vitreal face to supply the entire retina. This intricate mechanism was first described by Pettigrew and colleagues using fluorescein angiography to demonstrate the movement of molecules from the pecten to the very peripheral extremities of the retina with these small torsional movements of the globe [5].

There is no tapetum in the avian fundus, and hence the appearance is one dominated by the choroidal vasculature and pigmentation (Figure 9.10). Most species have a distinct fovea (Figure 9.11) where an increased density of photoreceptors gives increased visual resolution. Diurnal raptors and hummingbirds, among other species, have two foveolae (Figure 9.12) and it is suggest that in these bi-foveolate species one area is for high resolution distance vision while the other is for close work, such as manipulating prey when caught or positioning the beak very precisely as with the hummingbird. Some raptors such as the golden eagle have a concave, or more precisely convexiclivate fovea (Figure 9.13) allowing the image to fall on a much larger number of photoreceptors than

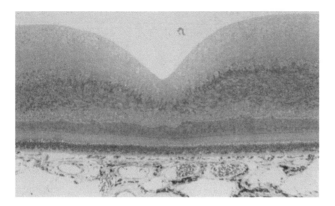

**Figure 9.13**   The convexiclivate fovea of the golden eagle.

possible if the fovea was flat and giving a much higher resolution than possible even with the human eye which we consider so highly evolved [6,7].

Another area in which birds supercede man's visual ability is in colour vision. While subprimate mammals have two-colour vision and might tempt us as trichromatic primates to consider ourselves as the pinnacle of ocular evolution, birds see not only in the three colours with which we are familiar but often in ultraviolet also. Birds have four types of cone peaks of light absoption of around 400 nm, 470 nm, 540 nm and 600 nm in the pigeon and 370 nm, 450 nm, 540 nm and 610 nm in the starling, to give just two examples (Figure 9.14). As well as having differently spectrally tuned photoreceptor pigments through changes in a few amino acids, avian photoreceptors also change their colour sensitivity with oil droplets of different colours. The three human cone photoreceptors have peak absorbances of 430 nm, 530 nm and 560 nm showing how avian colour vision includes wavelenths in the ultraviolet to which we are simply blind. Birds not only use their superior colour vision for food selection (probably the reason for trichromacy in primates seeking out ripe fruit in a leafy environment) but also for mate selection [8]. Casey Wood would have been delighted with such findings!

What such information should tell us is the importance of vision to birds and the great relevance of our attempts to correct visual disturbance in these individuals when presented to us with ocular abnormalities.

## What do birds see?

We are very fortunate in avian ophthalmology to have in Professor Graham Martin, a top class researcher who has devoted his professional career to the study of what birds see. From his doctoral studies on the visual acuity of tawny owls [9] to his most recent lucid review of avian binocular vision (or the lack of it) [10], he has provided an unparalleled appreciation of avian vision. But if one thing was to be taken from this

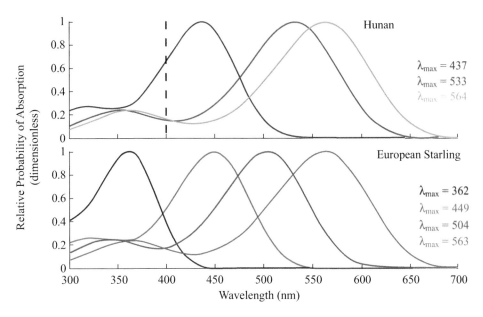

**Figure 9.14**   The four cone photoreceptors of the starling compared to the three of the human.

lifetime's work it should be that avian vision varies quite as much as the diversity of birds themselves. To try and group avocets, buzzards and crows together behaviourally not to mention owls, penguins and quail, would be quite ridiculous. And thus to try and pigeon-hole (if one will forgive the pun!) their vision into one description would be pointless. For birds' vision is intricately linked to their behaviour. The heron, which needs to visualise fish immediately under its beak, is bound to have very different vision from the kestrel which must focus on prey items moving hundreds of feet below it. To describe bird vision would take a whole book in itself – one which to my mind Professor Martin alone in the world of visual science is placed to write! And we might just add at this point that what appears obvious at a first glance – say for instance that the tawny owl has forward facing eyes with a wide field of binocular vision (Figure 9.15) – may turn out to be incorrect when subjected to critical analysis (Figure 9.16). Indeed Casey Wood realised that a century ago as shown by the diagrams in his *Fundus Oculi of Birds* (Figure 9.2). Thus we need to be very careful in what sweeping generalisations we make about avian vision. But having said that, barring a very few exceptions (the kiwi, for instance), birds have exceptional vision.

In those species for which refraction and visual acuity has been estimated, the American kestrel is emmetropic with an estimated acuity of 29 cycles/degree (cpd) when tested electrophysiologically, a method which those authors considered to underestimate acuity by some 37% in such species, giving them a final estimate of 46 cpd [11]. A study on the wedge-tailed eagle gave a maximum resolution acuity of between 132 and 146 cpd [12] with our average 20/20 vision equating to a paltry 30 cpd.

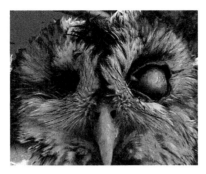

**Figure 9.15**   The forward facing eyes of the tawny owl. Here the frontal exposure has led to severe ulceration and scarring in the left eye and loss of the right following a road traffic accident.

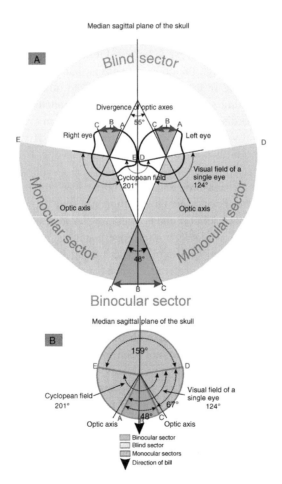

**Figure 9.16**   The true visual fields of the tawny owl, from *Binocularity* G Martin. Reproduced with permission from Professor Graham Martin.

# Evaluating the avian eye

As we noted in Chapter 3, the main problem with avian ophthalmology, as with eye examination of reptiles, amphibians and rodents – indeed most of the species covered in this volume – is the small size of the eye. Use of the direct ophthalmoscope is complicated by a tiny pupil in many species, but, with care, time and a close examination, full assessment is possible. The slit lamp biomicroscope can be really valuable in appreciating small lesions of the adnexa and anterior segment on its own and then the posterior segment can be viewed with a +30 D lens.

Because of the greater difficulty in performing a full ophthalmic examination, ancillary tests become even more valuable than in ophthalmoscopy of the dog or cat. Some do, however, have to be modified again because of the size of the eye. The Schirmer tear test strip, for instance, is just too wide to be placed in many avian eyes and, even if it were the right size, the amount of tears produced in a minute would not be sufficient to yield a measureable length of wetting. Two alternatives present themselves. One is to cut the strip of filter paper lengthways to halve its width [13]. The only problem with this is that we have little data for specific species of bird on what the normal wetting of a half-width test strip is. If only one eye is involved it may be possible to use the normal fellow eye as a control, although the concern there is that pathology in one eye alone may give a reactive increase in tearing in both eyes. The other alternative is to use a different measure of wetting such as the phenol red thread test. Here a yellow dye impregnated into a standardised cotton thread turns red when in contact with tears. Here we do have some normal values, reported for psittacines [14]. If values are not known for a specific species of bird, normal cage-mates can provide a useful set of normal values.

The same can be said for measurements of the intraocular pressure. Here the Tonopen applanation tonometer has been used most commonly and there are some reference values for different bird species, but if one is evaluating a species for which normal range of intraocular pressure is not available, normal cage-mates can be used to provide a reference range. The newer rebound Tonovet tonometer has the disadvantage that it has been used less frequently and so normal reference ranges are generally not available, but the great advantage that its tiny replaceable rebound tip can be used on corneas as small as 3 mm while the Tonopen tip requires a cornea around twice that wide. In the birds on which we have used the Tonovet we have not seen significantly different readings of intraocular pressure form those obtained with the Tonopen but those were birds with larger eyes and those results have as yet not been subjected to peer review in the veterinary literature.

Other ancilliary tests include cytology and bacteriology, again very useful additions to an ophthalmic examination given the proportion of diseases which may be infectious in nature. Cytology samples should be obtained with a cytobrush for immediate transfer to a clean glass microscope slide. Ideally bacteriology samples should be transferred straight from eye to suitable culture medium plate to avoid loss of organisms during transport. Polymerase chain reaction tests for other organisms can be very useful, especially considering the limited sample harvest which might be obtained from a small eye.

# Orbital disease

### Infraorbital and periocular sinusitis

#### Clinical signs

As noted above the proximity of the globe to the infraorbital sinus and particularly its diverticulum renders the eye prone to sinusitis. This can give exophthalmos or strabismus of the globe in acute phases, when infection and inflammation of the infraorbital sinus leads to a space-occupying lesion in the ventral orbit (Figure 9.17); enophthalmos is seen in chronic conditions where the sinus collapses because of fibrotic change after an acute infection (see Figure 9.24). Inflammation can lead to entrapment of air in the sinus giving a gas-filled mass periorbitally (Figure 9.18) while in other cases the sinus enlarges ventral to the globe distorting the palpebral aperture.

#### Aetiopathogenesis

Sometimes the infection gives rise to a solid caseous infected focus. The avian abscess, as is also the case in the reptile, is not the liquid purulent focus seen in mammals (which contains mostly neutrophils with their destructive enzymes). Instead, the avian abscess is a semi-solid lesion since the predominant cells are heterophils [15] which pave the way for fibrosis, to give what Professor John Cooper has suggested we call not an abscess but a fibriscess [16] (Figures 9.17 and 9.19).

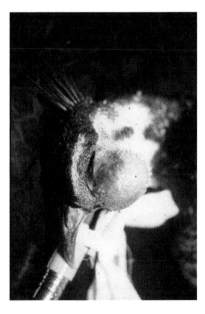

**Figure 9.17**   Infraorbital sinusitis with firm caseous swelling distorting the lower lid.

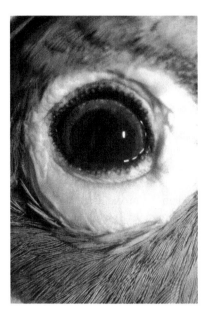

**Figure 9.18**   Entrapment of air in the infraorbital sinus in an Amazon parrot.

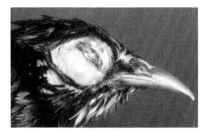

**Figure 9.19**   Distortion of the lid aperture from sinus pathology in a corvid (reproduced with permission from Dr Rudolf Korbel).

It may be that the problem is multifactorial with an infected blepharitis also present or hypovitaminosis A playing a part in the disease process and such possibilities should be taken into account in managing the case (see Figure 9.24).

## Clinical management

The potentially solid nature of such an infected focus means that one must be prepared to shell these lesions out of the infraorbital sinus through a skin incision below the lower eyelid. In such cases the problem may not be removing the inflammatory mass but reconstructing the stretched skin to ensure that the eyelid aperture still corresponds to the globe underneath. It may be, especially in the early stages, that the lesion is more fluid and in these cases irrigation of the entire cranial sinus system can be beneficial. In raptors with a profound sinusitis this can require holding the bird upsidedown and flush-

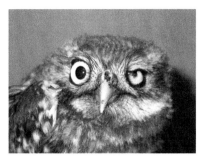

**Figure 9.20** Microphthalmos in a little owl.

ing saline through its nostrils to irrigate the far reaches of its sinus system. Systemic as well as local antibiotic after such a treatment regime is important and should be based on culture and sensitivity of samples taken during irrigation.

Chronic cases where enophthalmos occurs following collapse of the sinus can be very difficult to manage and topical antibiotic as well as systemic pain relief may be valuable in the management of the case, although cure is not possible.

### Microphthalmos and anophthalmos

#### Clinical signs

The presence of a small eye or indeed no apparent eye at all in the orbit signals microphthalmos or anophthalmos (Figure 9.20). Since the size of the globe defines the growth of the orbit, a bird with unilateral or bilateral microphthalmos may have an abnormally developed skull. Even so the orbit is often relatively over-large for the size of globe. In such cases a concurrent problem can be persistent conjunctivitis in the overly deep conjunctival sac. The eye itself may be normal but often microphthalmos is associated with other intraocular defects such as cataract or retinal dysplasia or detachment. It is important not to miss such findings in a small globe. Another possibility is related developmental defects in other body systems where a multisystem set of congenital defects may occur.

#### Aetiopathogenesis

Microphthalmos is a relatively common occurrence in birds of any species. There may well be a hereditary component to the condition but environmental influences in how the egg is managed before hatching can also be important. Birds thus affected normally have relatively poor vision but not often to the extent that their welfare in captivity is substantially compromised.

#### Clinical management

There is clearly nothing that can be done to resolve a congenital defect such as microphthalmos. Concurrent problems such as persistent conjunctivitis can be managed with topical antibiotic medication; cataract may conceivably be removed with phacoemulsification or irrigation/aspiration, although the concurrent presence of other ocular defects such as retinal dysplasia or detachment should be ruled out before surgery is attempted.

Anophthalmos, or what we might term extreme microphthalmos since a small ocular remnant is often found in the orbit, is clearly blinding when bilateral and chicks hatched without detectable eyes should be euthanased. Investigation of the status of eggs before hatching and the presence of the condition in related birds should be undertaken.

### Cryptophthalmos

Cryptophthalmos, where the globe is of normal size but hidden from view by constriction of the eyelid aperture can occur after injury or inflammation but is also seen in lutino colour-dilute cockatiels (Figure 9.21) [17]. The birds are rendered sightless by the extreme constriction of their eyelids. If surgery is performed to open the lid aperture, refibrosis occurs rapidly with considerable reduction in vision once more. These birds should not be bred from. A similar condition can occur in any bird after lid trauma (Figure 9.22), and again the eyelid appears to recicatrise after attempts to repair it.

Other congenital defects reported have included agenesis of part of the eyelid [18] and while surgical correction can be attempted, again the possibility of long-term damage to

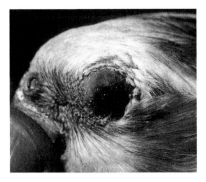

**Figure 9.21**   Cryptophthalmos in a cockatiel. (Reproduced courtesy of Dr N. Buyukmihci.)

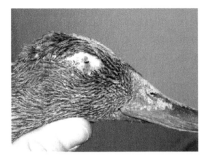

**Figure 9.22**   Cryptophthalmos after lid trauma in a mallard duck.

the ocular surface through inadequate protection during blinking may well suggest that euthanasia might be the kindest option in such cases.

## Lid and adnexal disease

### *Poxviral blepharitis*

#### *Clinical signs*

In different avian species poxvirus has quite different manifestations. In pigeons localised lid swelling with proliferative cutaneous growths is normally the predominant sign (Figure 9.23), although more severe lid swelling can cause ocular surface exposure in some birds (Figure 9.24). In psittacines a mild blepharitis with eyelid oedema and epiphora (Figure 9.25) develops into a more concerning condition with self-trauma causing lid ulceration (Figure 9.26) [19]. These lesions scab over and may develop to yield a mucopurulent discharge. The damaged lids may become sealed with a plug of inflammation or dry scabs. If not further injured by self-trauma the scabs can fall off in 2 weeks leaving mild scars. If further traumatic injury occurs, fibrosis of the scarred areas of lid can lead to an irregular eyelid margin with chronic corneal damage and blindness (Figure 9.27).

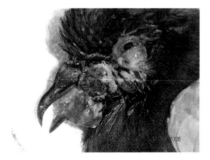

**Figure 9.23**   Proliferative poxviral lesions in a pigeon.

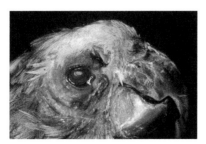

**Figure 9.24**   Exposure keratitis in poxvirus and hypovitaminosis A in an Amazon parrot.

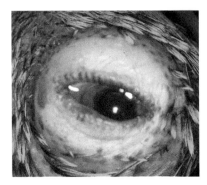

**Figure 9.25**  Eyelid oedema, blepharitis and epiphora in a pox-infected parrot.

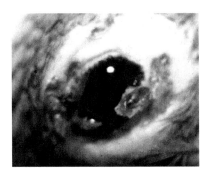

**Figure 9.26**  Traumatised lid in poxvirus-infected parrot.

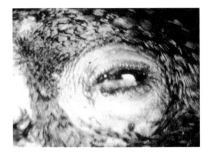

**Figure 9.27**  Chronic ocular surface damage with lid pathology in poxvirus infection.

### Aetiopathogenesis

There are three strains of avian poxvirus, the pigeon, canary and fowl (poultry) variants, of which the canary strain is seen most commonly in captive pscittacines. The different strains in different bird species give substantially different results as noted above. Avian pox can be a very damaging infection of the adnexa either because of the proliferative lesions or more commonly from self-trauma which leaves ulcerated areas prone to further scab formation and a vicious circle of self-trauma and irritation. This was particularly the case when large consignments of parrots were transported in crates from the Amazon to be kept as captive individuals in North America and Europe [20]. The stocking density of birds increased the likelihood of poxviral transmission between birds and the stress of capture and transport crippled their immune system rendering them much more susceptible to infection. In mild infections, however, where good-quality care is available at the time of infection the initial lesions can resolve well.

### Clinical management

The key factor in successful treatment of periocular poxviral disease is prevention of self-trauma. Use of a thin plastic collar to prevent the bird's claws reaching the periocular region can lead to considerable suffering and stress for the bird. A better option is the use of a dilute baby shampoo around the lids, taking care not to apply any to the ocular surface. This softens the scabs, renders them less irritating and also less likely to be torn off by self-trauma. Antiviral medication is not generally considered effective against poxviral infection in birds.

## Hypovitaminosis A

### Clinical signs

Vitamin A deficiency can give rise to periocular and conjunctival swelling with ocular discharge (Figure 9.24). The problem with these as signs of deficiency is that they may also occur in diseases such as poxvirus blepharitis or sinusitis. Thus hypovitaminosis must always be considered as a contributory factor when these periocular signs are seen. As this is a systemic condition, ocular signs will often be accompanied by white plaques in and around the mouth, laboured and open-mouth breathing, sometimes profuse nasal discharge together with sneezing or, in other cases, dry crusted external nares. Dermal dyskeratosis and feather abnormalities may also be seen.

### Aetiopathogenesis

Vitamin A is a key molecule regulating normal epithelial growth. Thus deficiency leads to skin, feather and mucous membrane abnormalities, which is particularly noticeable and potentially damaging around the eye. As noted above deficiency, even at a subclinical level, can be an important contributory factor to other periocular diseases.

### Clinical management

The clinical presentation of a bird with signs as noted above should always lead first to a thorough history taking focusing on the nutritional status of the animal. Use of a seed-based diet, especially one with sunflower seeds, is highly suggestive of a dietary deficiency of a fat-soluble vitamin like vitamin A. A suggestive history and appropriate clinical signs are generally sufficient for a tentative diagnosis of a deficiency without the need for measuring serum levels of the vitamin. While changing the dietary regime is clearly the long-term aim, this can be difficult in the short term as these birds are as good as addicted to these high-energy seeds. Injectable vitamin A can be valuable, although one must ensure that hypervitaminosis A is not provoked. Oral beta carotene can be a safer option from this perspective. The key factor in immediate ocular management is care of the periorbital area with a lubricative antibiotic gel.

### *Knemidokoptes infection*

#### *Clinical signs*

The mite *Knemidokoptes pilae*, commonly associated with the conditions podoknemi-dokoptes (scaly leg or tassel-foot) [21] and similar proliferative lesions around the beak (scaly-face or tassel-beak), can cause substantial tissue outgrowths around the eye (Figure 9.28 and Figure 9.29). The findings are pathognomonic for the mite infestation.

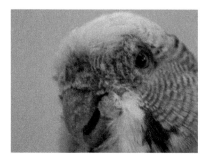

**Figure 9.28**   *Knemidicoptes pilae* infection giving proliferative periocular lesions.

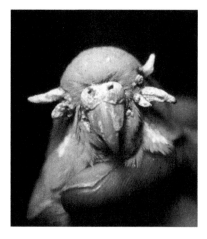

**Figure 9.29**   *Knemidicoptes pilae* infection giving periocular 'tassels'.

### Aetiopathogenesis

The mite burrows into the cornified epithelium around the eyelids and provokes a variable, but sometimes marked, proliferative reaction. This often looks disfiguring and alarming to the owner but rarely causes much discomfort to the affected bird, although trauma can cause tissue damage with bleeding on occasion.

### Clinical management

Treatment with ivermectin at a dose of 200 µg/kg by intramuscular injection once weekly for three treatments has been effective in one previous report [22], and by a single dose in another [23], although neither of these cases were periocular. Softening the proliferative lesions with paraffin oil is said by some to prevent irritation but in this author's experience these lesions are not markedly pruritic.

## Lid neoplasia

### Clinical signs

Neoplasms in the avian eyelid are rare while non-neoplastic swellings, either cystic or inflammatory from sinusitis are much more common. Thus any periocular swelling, while it may be cancerous, is more likely to be non-neoplastic [24]. Cystic swellings or those resulting from sinusitis are generally, in this author's experience at least, more likely to be smooth rather than verrucose in their surface appearance as shown in the virally induced papilloma in Figure 9.30.

### Aetiopathogenesis

Clearly any neoplasm can arise de novo without a specific aetiological agency. Thus lymphosarcoma [25] and chondrosarcoma [26] appear in the literature but many other tumours are likely to go unreported.

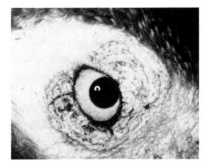

**Figure 9.30** Viral papillomata in an African grey parrot. Reproduced with permission from Professor Elliott Jacobson.

## Clinical management

Eyelid surgery to remove neoplastic masses can be performed but the small size of the eye and thin nature of the periocular skin mean that such surgery should be perfomed under an operating microscope by someone well versed in microsurgical techniques.

## Conjunctivitis

### Clinical signs

The classic features of any inflammation are hyperaemia, swelling, discharge and pain and conjunctivitis is no different. Thus we will see conjunctival hyperaemia, chemosis (conjunctival oedema), ocular discharge, either serous or mucopurulent depending on the involvement or otherwise of bacteria, and also blepharospasm indicating discomfort, a part of ocular inflammation which is often forgotten [27].

### Aetiopathogenesis

We can differentiate avian conjunctivitis into three distinct groups. First are those conditions which are specifically localised – foreign bodies or conjunctival infections. Secondly are those where the conjunctivitis is a manifestation of periocular disease, these predominantly involving sinusitis as covered above. The third group is those cases in which the conjunctivitis occurs concurrent with a systemic disease, with the link between the two normally involving septicaemia.

A surprising number of birds can be affected by foreign bodies – in one report of free ranging red-shouldered hawks 7% of them had grass florets lodged behind their third eyelid. In pet birds foreign bodies such a millet seeds, seed husks and feathers may also be seen associated with foreign body conjunctivitis. The infectious organisms involved with this first group range from Gram-positive and Gram-negative flora, *Chlamydophila* and *Mycoplasma*, fungi such as *Cryptosporidium* and even mycobacteria such as *M. avium* [28]. In pigeons the 'one-eyed cold' is a general term for conjunctivitis which can often be related to *Chlamydophila* or *Mycoplasma* infection.

But we must note that merely finding an organism in a conjunctival sac does not make it the cause of the lesion. What of the bacteria isolated from normal eyes? Work on the normal microbiological flora of the avian conjunctiva showed that 71% of the captive exotic birds sampled had at least one bacterial isolate from their conjunctival sac [29]. Eighty-six percent of these were staphylococcal species or *Corynebacterium* while Gram-negative bacteria were isolated from 14% of birds and fungi from 9%. In another study 59% of sampled birds showed a bacterial isolate and 50% of these were Gram-positive cocci [30].

Finding a profuse growth of a single organism is good evidence that it may well be a causative agent. Clearly it is not possible to fulfil Koch's postulates for each case of infection we come across, but the finding of a profuse growth of a single bacterium is much better evidence than a scanty growth of two or more isolates.

Having said that Crispin and Barnett recovered *Escherichia coli* from the majority of clinically normal ducklings and considered that the neonatal flora in these birds were derived from the intestinal flora [31]. *Chlamydophila psittaci* is frequently isolated from

Australian parakeets with keratoconjunctivitis and from conjunctivitis in pigeons and finches [32]. *Mycoplasma* is more often isolated from pigeons with conjunctivitis, the so-called one-eyed cold, although as we noted above *Chlamydophila* can cause this as can *Salmonella*.

Parasitic conjunctivitis has been reported with the nematode *Oxyspirura mansoni* in cockatoos with epiphora. The worm lives in the lower conjunctival sac and sometimes the nasolacrimal duct which it uses to reach the eye from the crop. The worm requires a cockroach as its intermediate host, so birds kept inside are unlikely to be affected [33]. *Thelazia* nematodes have also been noted causing conjunctivitis in birds although they are more normally parasites of mammalian hosts [34]. Tremadode flukes of the genus *Philophthalmus* have been reported as causing conjunctivitis in a number of avian species [35].

## Clinical management

The first step in investigating avian conjunctivitis then, must be to evaluate which of these three groups the conjunctivitis falls. Is it associated with localised infection or a foreign body? Is it part of a condition such as sinusitis, or is there a more systemic component with the bird more dull and lethargic and showing other clinical signs of generalised infection?

First a history must be taken. Are any other in-contact birds affected or maybe a new unquarantined cage-mate? Is the bird exposed to a noxious stimulus such as cigarette smoke or perhaps the carpets have just been cleaned with a proprietary product? A close ophthalmic examination is of course required but ensure that careful assessment is made of areas which might not be covered on a cursory examination such as the conjunctival sac behind the third eyelid – all too often this is where a foreign body can lie unrecognised. Third a full clinical examination is mandatory, focusing particularly on the upper respiratory tract but taking care to note any other possible infectious foci.

After this clinical assessment come ancilliary tests – first a Schirmer tear test to determine degree of tear production and then cytology, bacteriology and PCR sample collection for possible infectious agents. Bacterial infection is the most commonly reported cause of conjunctivitis, so topical antibiotic is suggested even before bacteriological results are obtained. Recrudescence occurs often because concurrent sinus infection is also seen so systemic antibiosis is important in addition to topical treatment, with a broad-spectrum agent advisable. Use of tetracycline or fluoroquinolone is recommended given the likelihood that *Mycoplasma* or *Chlamydophila* may be involved in many cases of conjunctivitis. In cases where fungal elements are seen and agents such as *Candida* or *Aspergillus* isolated, topical treatment with amphotericin B at 4% has been advised as oral dosing is not tolerated well. Where systemic medication is required 5-fluorocytosine has been suggested orally at 400 mg/kg per day in divided doses [18].

## Cockatiel conjunctivitis

### Clinical signs

Specific note should be made of conjunctivitis which causes quite profound chemosis and hyperaemia predominantly in cockatiels but also in budgerigars [36]. There is

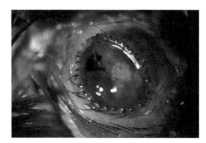

**Figure 9.31**   Chemotic and hyperaemic conjunctivitis in a cockatiel.

hyperaemia, chemosis and a clear watery discharge (Figure 9.31). Some of the birds thus affected also have neurological signs such as partial lid paresis and reduced jaw tone. Many of these birds also have intestinal *Giardia* infection and respond to treatment with metronidazole and vitamin E.

### Aetiopathogenesis

To date no organism has been isolated from the eyes of birds with this condition although given the response of the condition to topical chlortetracycline one assumes that either *Chlamydophila* or *Mycoplasma* may be responsible.

### Clinical managemernt

Use of topical chlortetracycline resolves the vast majority of these cases. Once the ocular signs are resolving, showing that this is indeed the correct course of therapy, the bird should be dosed with systemic tetracycline, since if ocular tissues are affected, it is highly likely that organisms will also be found in the nasopharynx. Currently the standard topical chlortetracycline in the UK, Aureomycin, is not available, and in its place topical fluoroquinolones such as ofloxacin (Exocin, Allergan) may be effective.

## Lovebird eye disease

### Clinical signs

This condition again manifests as conjunctivitis and periorbital swelling with blepharitis and serous ocular discharge leading to hyperaemia and ulceration of the region and the serous discharge becoming mucopurulent with concurrent bacterial infection. The disease here is more severe than those previously mentioned in that generalised depression is seen with lethargy, anorexia and commonly death within a few days.

### Aetiopathogenesis

No specific infectious agent has been isolated from affected birds although histological evaluation has shown inclusions in conjunctival cells and sometimes also proliferative inflammatory lesions with lymphoid infiltrates and subepithelial oedema. Stress is probably an important factor in the initiation of the disease, as transport and the introduction of new cage-mates into the environment have been reported as being associated with outbreaks of the disease.

### Clinical management

Isolation of affected birds is important both to reduce the stress on the bird itself, whose cage-mates have been reported to be aggressive towards affected individuals, and also for in-contact birds in case an infectious cause is at the root of the problem.

# Corneal disease

## Corneal ulceration

### Clinical signs

Blepharospasm, epiphora and signs of self-trauma are often the first signs of corneal ulceration in a bird (Figure 9.32). Ophthalmic examination reveals an area of the ocular surface giving an irregular reflection of a light shone onto it. The ulcer margin, either crisp and sharp in a recent ulcer or maybe ragged and irregular in a chronic non-healing one, is often evident on examination with some magnification from a direct ophthalmoscope at +20 D or a slit lamp biomicroscope.

Fluorescein can be very valuable in demarcating the extent of an ulcer and also for determining whether the edge of the surrounding epithelium is adherent to the underlying basement membrane and stroma or is devitalised and non-adherent, as in corneal epithelial basement membrane dystrophy or so-called boxer ulcers in dogs.

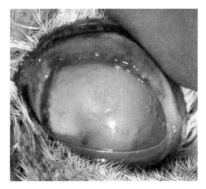

**Figure 9.32** Chronic corneal ulceration in an aged snowy owl. Note that chronic lid pathology here probably contributes to the non-healing nature of the ulcer in addition to the age of the bird.

### Aetiopathogenesis

As with any species, the majority of avian corneal ulceration occurs secondary to trauma, either from an external source such as a foreign body or from what we might call an internal agency, such as a swollen irregular eyelid abrading the ocular surface. More chronic non-healing ulcers can often be seen in older birds, where epithelial healing is not as rapid and complete as in a younger animal. Some birds also seem to have a basement membrane dystrophy-like lesion where the epithelial edge is non-adherent.

### Clinical management

A superficial erosion subsequent to localised trauma in a normal healthy cornea should heal within 1 week. The normal flow of epithelial cells from the stem cell population at the limbus, across the cornea as a basal epithelial cell and then up through the layers of the stratified squamous epithelium, becoming wing cells and then squames and finally desquamating at the corneal surface ensures that epithelial erosions should heal within this short time. The question is should a prophylactic antibiotic be used topically to ensure that bacterial infection does not supervene? It would seem only reasonable to attempt to stop invading organisms from crossing this denuded and thus at-risk area of ocular surface. Yet it is likely that by giving antibiotic we are actually killing the normal commensal flora and thus may be leaving a path open for pathogenic bacteria to take over the binding sites normally occupied by these comensals. And yet perhaps the one corneal ulcer you decide to leave without antibiotic will be the one that develops a *Pseudomonas* infection and begins to melt, with collagenases from the bacteria destroying the otherwise healthy stroma beneath the ulcer surface.

It may be that the antibiotic or, more likely, the preservatives and stabilisers in such topical medications, may themselves slow ulcer healing, but given the horrendous results of true pathogenic bacterial colonisation of a corneal ulcer, it is probably correct to use an antibiotic prophylactically in corneal ulcers in birds. What we should say is that the antibiotic to chose should be one that is more likely to kill the Gram-negative pathogens on a corneal surface than the Gram-positive commensals.

In deep ulcers or ones that show signs of beginning to melt, that is to say those with an irregular oedematous surface, topical autologous serum should be used frequently. The serum contains TIMPs, tissue inhibitors of the matrix metalloproteinases (MMPs) which are causing the collagen breakdown manifest as corneal melting. Serum, or indeed plasma, with EDTA added also has the advantage that the EDTA chelates calcium which is required by many MMPs and thus reduces their activity.

A long-standing non-healing but sterile ulcer may benefit from ocular surface protection using a tarsorrhaphy simply fashioned by placing two 4/0 vicryl sutures to close the lids. This is to be preferred to a third eyelid flap, for the powerful muscles that draw the third eyelid across the ocular surface may well pull the sutures through the margin of the third eyelid, with a failure of corneal protection and further damage to the ocular adnexa.

## Amazon keratitis

### Clinical signs

A transient corneal inflammation with a subtle punctate appearance has been reported in Central American Amazon parrots [37]. The lesions generally begin in the medial cornea, extend across the ocular surface and then resolve, normally within 1 week. The surface lesions are transiently fluorescein positive and are seldom more than an epithelial erosion. On occasion the lesion extends more deeply in the stroma with associated uveitic change giving either a dull-appearing iris or occasionally a more severe inflammation with fibrin clots and synechiae. Some birds develop a concurrent sinusitis.

### Aetiopathogenesis

These lesions have been noted associated with capture in the wild and transportation. Their development may merely be one associated with damage to the cornea during capture complicated by capture and transport-related stress.

### Clinical management

Neither topical antibiotics nor antivirals have been found to improve the course of the disease significantly. Most lesions self-heal within one week but animals should be examined regularly to ensure that no complicating factors lead to worsening of lesions rather than their healing. If lesions are worsening, supportive care with topical antibiotics would be indicated.

## Mynah bird keratitis

### Clinical signs

Corneal erosions are common in caged birds especially after capture and transport. The vast majority of these heal within 48 hours through the natural migration of corneal epithelial cells from the stem cell population at the limbus. Mynah birds seem prone to more severe and long-lasting handling-related traumatic corneal lesions. In one study 96% of birds examined immediately after shipping were noted to have corneal epithelial erosions with associated blepharospasm and some conjunctival hyperaemia [38].

### Aetiopathogenesis

As with the Amazon punctate keratitis discussed above, most of these lesions resolve with 1 week, but some leave corneal scarring and permanent opacity. Other birds develop chronic keratoconjunctivitis with conjunctival masses, widespread corneal ulceration and neovascularisation. In several of these severely affected birds systemic aspergillosis may be an important factor in causing immunosuppression. In others, herpetic keratitis, responsive to acyclovir, has been suggested as a complicating factor.

### Clinical management

As with the Amazon keratitis above supportive care is probably all that is needed in many cases of mynah keratitis, but tear replacement, topical antibiosis and antiviral therapy where required should be considered.

## Uveal disease

### Clinical signs

The classical signs of uveitis are a miotic pupil, inflammatory changes in the anterior segment from aqueous flare through to keratitic precipitates of cells from the aqueous onto the posterior corneal face, and in severe cases frank hypopyon (Figure 9.33). Veterinarians will have noted such changes in cats and dogs with uveitis and the same signs are seen in birds with uveitis. Many birds have only the mildest signs with flare reducing the clarity of iris detail and the pupil margin, while other more severe cases may have purulent material or haemorrhage in the anterior chamber. Chronic mild uveitis may result merely in a darkened hyperpigmented iris (Figure 9.34). In more severe cases, often after trauma, posterior synechiae are seen (Figure 9.35). When these adhesions between iris and anterior lens capsule prevent aqueous passage through the pupil, glaucoma can supervene.

### Aetiopathogenesis

Corneal disease can lead to uveitis when severe, probably through an antidromal trigeminal stimulation causing breakdown of the blood–aqueous barrier with subsequent liberation of fibrin and leucocytes into the aqueous humour. Another cause of uveitis in birds is association with systemic infectious disease. Here again blood–aqueous barrier disrup-

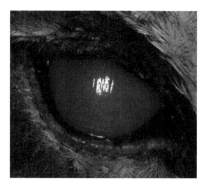

**Figure 9.33**   Severe hypopyon filling the anterior segment in a uveitic tawny owl.

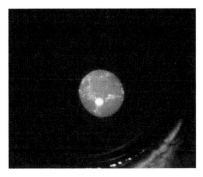

**Figure 9.34** Lens-induced uveitis with a dull dark iris with mature cataract in a Harris hawk.

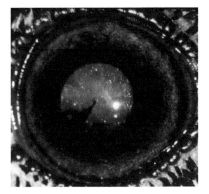

**Figure 9.35** Post-traumatic cataract and uveitis with synechia.

tion is important. Bilateral uveitis has been reported in a lovebird with staphylococcal septicaemia [39], while psittacines with reovirus infection showed disseminated intravascular coagulation and associated uveitis [40]. Some had hypopyon, some intraocular haemorrhage and most recovered but with synechiae.

Ocular trauma in any bird species, but seen most particularly in raptors, can result in uveitis. A final cause of uveitis is the dissemination of lens protein into the anterior chamber either acutely through lens capsule rupture after trauma or more chronically associated with mature cataract formation. Ingress of water into the capsular bag of the lens results in enlargement of the lens. This causes microfractures of the lens capsule with concomitant release of soluble lens proteins into the aqueous. The story here runs that the iris has not encountered these proteins previously, as they have been trapped in the lens until now. Release of this antigen, novel to the intraocular immune system, results in an immune activation and resulting uveitis. This neat story is probably rather too simple – lens proteins are not necessarily hidden from the neighbouring uveal lymphocytes prior to such release but it is probably the level of their presence after cataract maturity which leads to uveitic change.

## Clinical management

The classic treatment of uveitis in mammals involves mydriasis and anti-inflammatory medication. Topical steroids such as prednisolone acetate and/or non-steroidals like ketorolac or flurbiprofen work in birds just as well as in mammals, but the striated muscle of the iris means that atropine will not work to dilate the avian pupil. While it takes relatively little non-depolarising muscle relaxant such as vecuronium to dilate a normal pupil, in an inflamed iris frequent dosing is needed to produce adequate mydriasis, and intracemeral suxamethonium (i.e. drug injected into the anterior chamber) may be required. The trouble here is that overdosing with potential systemic paralytic effects can be all too easily a potentially fatal side effect.

# Lens disease

## Cataracts

### Clinical signs

One of the most common conditions seen in the avian eye is cataract (Figure 9.34). By the time many birds are presented to the veterinarian they will have a total mature white cataract. Evaluation of the lens with more subtle changes can be readily achieved with the direct ophthalmoscope set at +10 D, although often a slit lamp biomicroscope can give a better view of lens pathology in these very small eyes. Other ocular signs of importance when evaluating a cataract include assessing the iris for lens-induced uveitis, when there will be a dull dark homogeneous hue to the iris face (Figure 9.34), and retinal detachment, which may occur in mature or hypermature cataract and can really only be determined by ocular ultrasonography when the cataract is mature or nearly so.

### Aetiopathogenesis

A common cause of cataracts in birds is trauma, whether in wild or captive individuals (Figure 9.35). Others are age-related, seen in older birds (Figure 9.36) Some cataracts

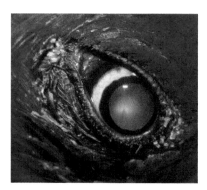

**Figure 9.36**   Age-related cataract in a 48-year-old macaw.

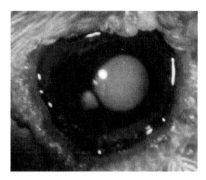

**Figure 9.37**  Inherited cataract in a Norwich canary.

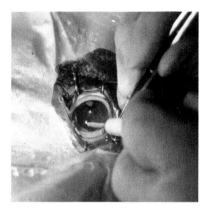

**Figure 9.38**  Phacoemulsification of a cataract in an owl.

are inherited – that seen in the Norwich canary (Figure 9.37) is one such and thus related birds should always be examined if possible. Given that psittacine species can have long life expectancies, age-related cataract is not uncommon [41]. A deficiency in dietary antioxidants and daylight, which accounts for much of the age-related cataract seen in humans, may be important in older birds. Drugs and diabetes are factors noted in man but as yet their importance is unclear in birds. Indeed the majority of lens opacities seen in birds are post-traumatic, although, as a greater number of older birds are examined, we might expect idiopathic age-related cataract to be recognised more frequently.

## Clinical management

The only curative treatment for cataract is surgery. Phacoemulsification can be used in larger eyes but where this is not possible irrigation and aspiration with an irrigation/aspiration handpiece or even with a needle can be employed given the soft nature of the majority of birds' lenses (Figure 9.38) [42]. Cases with lens-induced or post-tramatic uveitis should be rigorously managed with topical steroid drops up to five times daily to ensure that the intraocular inflammation is controlled as well as possible. Indeed this

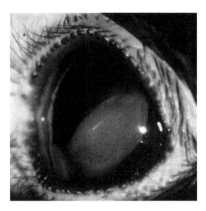

**Figure 9.39**  Lens luxation in a hybrid hawk.

highlights the fact that only birds that can be easily handled might be seen as appropriate for surgery given the frequency of topical drops required for several weeks before and after the surgery.

### Lens luxation

#### Clinical signs

Displacement of the lens is seen with surprising frequency in birds and is evident normally because of the aphakic crescent evident when the lens has deviated ventrally, its zonule having been disrupted (Figure 9.39). In many cases, given the pathogenesis noted below, there will be concurrent ocular abnormalities, either resulting from the trauma that luxated the lens in the first place, or the mature or hypermature cataract, often with resulting lens-induced uveitis. In such cases it can be difficult to differentiate these two aetiopathological paths and the taking of a history, if available, is crucial.

#### Aetiopathogenesis

The majority of luxated lenses are seen after trauma, although the changes in a maturing cataract rendering it more spherical can lead to tension on the zonule with its rupture and subsequent lens luxation. This is more seen in birds with large eyes such as owls rather than in small birds where the lens is already spherical to maximise its focusing power in such small eyes.

#### Clinical managment

In many cases the bird is not unduly concerned about the lens luxation. If there is little inflammation it may be best to leave the lens in place in this author's opinion, although its removal by phacoemulsification is certainly possible; alternatively it may be removed by means of an intracapsular lendectomy, if the size of the eye does not permit use of a phacoemulsification handpiece [43,44].

## Retinal disease

### Clinical signs

Much avian retinal disease is trauma-related and thus clinical signs include in the short term detachment and haemorrhage, often with damage to the pecten (Figure 9.40 and Figure 9.41) [45]. Focal pigmented areas are seen in some owls and have been associated with sunlight exposure in some reports and toxoplasmosis in others. This author consid-

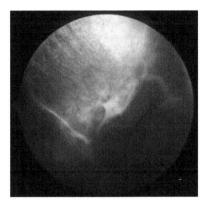

**Figure 9.40**   Inflammatory change around a damaged pecten in an aged eagle owl.

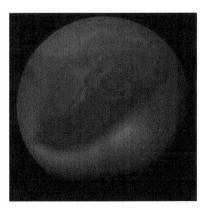

**Figure 9.41**   Persistent haemorrhage from a damaged pecten in a tawny owl.

ers that they may well be a normal variant, as they are seen in numerous raptors and not associated with concurrent posterior segment inflammation [46].

### Aetiopathogenesis

Again the predominant cause of retinal disease in birds appears to be trauma. Reports of inherited retinal degenerations so common in dogs are vanishingly rare in birds, presumably because they have not been looked for and techniques such as electroretinography are only available for birds in a small number of specialist centres. The size of the bird eye again is a limiting factor with wire electrodes needing to be used and the minute voltages produced requiring very substantial amplification against what is, relatively speaking, a noisy electrical background. Thus photoreceptor dysplasia has been reported in pigeons [47] and raptors [48] and a retinal defect leading to globe enlargement has been evaluated in detail in one line of chickens, clinically [49], histopathologically [50], and by electroretinography [51]. While these can hardly been considered pet birds, the techniques used can equally be employed in birds in any captive environment, and thus reference is made to them here. Retinal degeneration has been reported in a psittacine [52], but the majority of retinal disease reported in the veterinary literature is traumatic or infectious in origin. *Toxoplasma* has been reported to have caused histopathological chorioretinal lesions in one group of canaries in the same way that it can in people [53] and blindness in a different group of the same species in an earlier report [54]; we have shown, however, that there was no serological evidence for *Toxoplasma* infection in similar lesions in a small sample of owls [45]. Here trauma was the underlying cause of retinal detachment.

## Horner's syndrome

### Clinical signs

The classic triad of miosis, ptosis and enophthalmos is not seen in birds with sympathetic denervation the eye. To start with the iris sphincter and dilator muscles are not autonomically innervated and thus we are not dealing with miosis with this condition in birds. The globe is much less mobile in the avian orbit and thus one does not see enophthalmos and third eyelid protrusion. The only sign left is ptosis, and this is an eyelid paresis that can be reversed with topical dilute phenylephrine (Figure 9.42 and Figure 9.43) [55,56].

### Aetiopathogenesis

In the two reported cases of avian Horner's syndrome an aetiology was not given; as so often with unexplained lesions in raptors, trauma is invoked as the most likely cause.

### Clinical management

Unless further evaluation with radiography and ultrasonography is used in an attempt to locate the cause of the sympathetic dysfunction these cases, no further diagnostic or

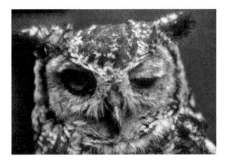

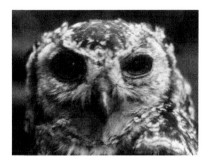

**Figure 9.42** Horner's syndrome in an African eagle owl.

**Figure 9.43** The bird in Figure 9.42 after administration of topical phenylephrine.

therapeutic measures are required. The birds are not unduly compromised by this condition and treatment is not possible.

## Enucleation

A number of reports exist for various ocular surgeries in birds from operations for entropion, for cataract and for lens luxation already discussed above [33–35,57], to corneal reconstructive surgery after trauma [58], or even corneal grafting [59]. Given the high incidence of trauma, enucleation is the most common ocular surgery in birds, yet it can be difficult to undertake because of the scleral ossicles which can preclude removing the eye without collapsing it. Two alternatives have been reported. First a very useful technique of enlarging the palpebral aperture by joining it to the aural meatus has been published (Figure 9.44) which allows the entire globe to be removed even in owls with tubular eyes [60]. Secondly evisceration, where the intraocular contents are removed and the resulting space filled with a conforming sterile padding, is possible (Figure 9.45) [61,62]. The problem with enucleation is that, as we saw at the beginning of this chapter in Figures 9.2 and 9.4, the globe takes up a significant proportion of the avian skull in terms of volume and weight. Enucleation is not only difficult, it may leave the bird unbalanced after surgery. Evisceration opens the cornea, removes the intraocular contents and then, following removal of the palpebral margins, closes the lid skin over the resulting blind and pain-free globe.

This leaves us with one final question: if vision is so central to a bird's telos – its very reason for being – is removing an eye an appropriate surgery to be doing? Should a unilaterally anophthalmic bird, or even one bilaterally blind after trauma or disease, be kept alive? Professor Martin's paper [9] puts binocularity in a new light and suggests that maybe after all birds do not necessarily need two eyes to fulfil their life's requirements. While reports of successful reintroduction into the wild of uniocular birds are not common, they do occur, showing that release after adequate training might be appropriate [63].

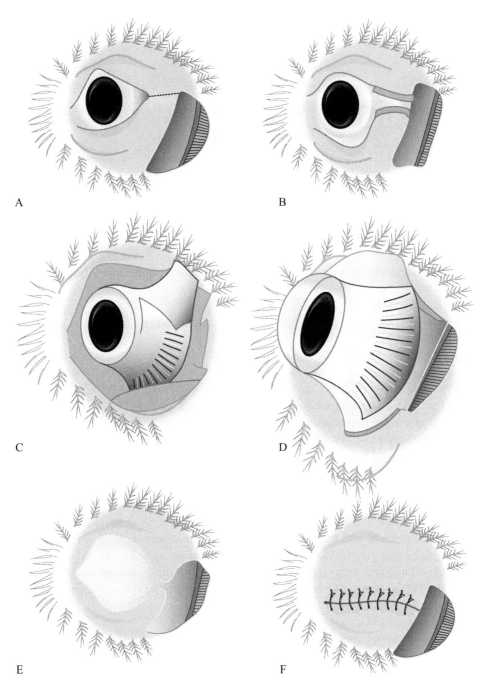

A

B

C

D

E    F

**Figure 9.44**   Enucleation via enlargement of the palpebral aperture through the aural meatus, redrawn after Murphy *et al.* 1983. An incision joins the lateral canthus to the aural meatus, enlarging the aperture through which the tubular globe can be removed after careful resection, with the resulting cavity closed with permanent sutures.

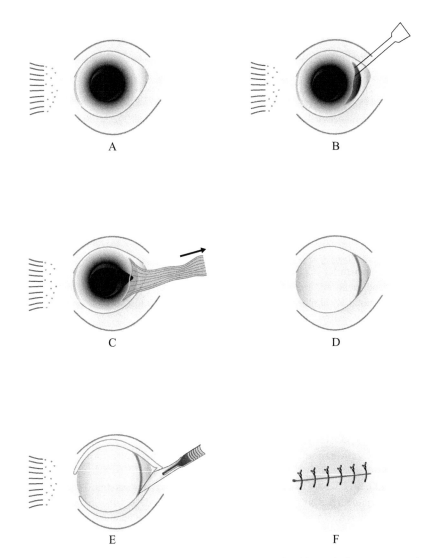

**Figure 9.45**   Evisceration of the globe as a potentially preferable technique compared to full enucleation. The cornea is incised and intraocular contents removed by traction. The cornea is removed and the globe packed with haemostatic gauze. The lid margins are resected and sutured to close the skin over the open globe.

## References

1. Martin GR. Eye. In: AS King, J McLelland, eds. *Form and Function in Birds*, vol. 3. London: Academic Press, 1985.
2. Willis AM, Wilkie DA. Avian ophthalmology: part 1: anatomy, examination and diagnostic techniques. J Avian Med Surg 1999;13:160–166 and part 2: review of ophthalmic diseases. J Avian Med Surg 1999;13:245–251.
3. Ott M. Visual accommodation in vertebrates: mechanisms, physiological response and stimuli. J Comp Physiol A 2006;192: 97–111.

4. Sivak J G. Avian mechanisms for vision in air and water. Trends Neurosci 1980;12: 314–317.

5. Pettigrew JD, Wallman J, Wildsoet CF. Saccadic oscillations facilitate ocular perfusion from the avian pecten. Nature 1990;343:362–363.

6. Fite KV, Rosenfield-Wessels S. A comparative study of deep avian foveas. Brain Behav Evol 1975;12:97–115.

7. Locket NA. Problems of deep foveas. Aust N Z J Ophthalmol 1992;20:281–295.

8. Bennett AT, Cuthill IC, Partridge JC, Lunau K. Ultraviolet plumage colors predict mate preferences in starlings. Proc Natl Acad Sci U S A 1997;94:8618–8621.

9. Martin GR, Gordon IE. Visual acuity in the tawny owl (*Strix aluco*). Vision Res 1974;14: 1393–1397.

10. Martin GR. What is binocular vision for? A birds' eye view. J Vis 2009;9:14.1–19.

11. Gaffney MF, Hodos W. The visual acuity and refractive state of the American kestrel (*Falco sparverius*). Vision Res 2003;43:2053–2059.

12. Reymond L. Spatial visual acuity of the eagle *Aquila audax*: a behavioural, optical and anatomical investigation. Vision Res 1985;25:1477–1491.

13. Korbel R, Leitenstorfer P. [The modified Schirmer tear test in birds – a method for checking lacrimal gland function]. Tierarztl Prax Ausg K Klientiere Heimtiere 1998;26:284–294.

14. Holt E, Rosenthal K, Shofer FS. The phenol red thread tear test in large psittaciformes. Vet Ophthalmol 2006;9:109–113.

15. Montali RJ. Comparative pathology of inflammation in the higher vertebrates (reptiles, birds and mammals) J Comp Pathol 1988;99:1–26.

16. Huchzermeyer FW, Cooper JE. Fibriscess, not abscess, resulting from a localised inflammatory response to infection in reptiles and birds. Vet Rec 2000;147:515–517.

17. Buyukmihci NC, Murphy CJ, Paul-Murphy J, Hacker DV, Laratta LJ, Brooks DE. Eyelid malformation in four cockatiels. J Am Vet Med Assoc 1990;196:1490–1492.

18. Kern TJ, Murphy CJ, Heck WR. Partial upper eyelid agenesis in a peregrine falcon. J Am Vet Med Assoc 1985;187:1207.

19. McDonald SE, Lowenstine LJ, Ardans AA. Avian pox in blue-fronted Amazon parrots. J Am Vet Med Assoc 1981;179:1218–1222.

20. Karpinski LG, SL Clubb. Clinical aspects of ophthalmology in caged birds. In: RW Kirk, ed. *Current Veterinary Therapy IX*. Philadelphia, PA: WB Saunders, 1986; pp. 616–621.

21. Pence DB, Cole RA, Brugger KE, Fischer JR. Epizootic podoknemidokoptiasis in American robins. J Wildl Dis 1999;35:1–7.

22. Miller DS, Taton-Allen GF, Campbell TW. Knemidokoptes in a Swainson's hawk, *Buteo swainsoni*. J Zoo Wildl Med 2004;35:400–402.

23. Schulz TA, Stewart JS, Fowler ME. Knemidokoptes mutans (Acari: Knemidocoptidae) in a great-horned owl (*Bubo virginianus*). J Wildl Dis 1989;25:430–432.

24. Jacobson ER, Mladinich CR, Clubb S, Sundberg JP, Lancaster WD. Papilloma-like virus infection in an African gray parrot. J Am Vet Med Assoc 1983;183:1307–1308.

25. Ramos-Vara JA, Smith EJ, Watson GL. Lymphosarcoma with plasmacytoid differentiation in a scarlet macaw (*Ara macao*). Avian Dis 1997;41:499–504.

26. Spalding MG, Woodard JC. Chondrosarcoma in a wild great white heron from southern Florida. J Wildl Dis 1992;28:151–153.

27. Abrahams GA, Paul-Murphy J, Murphy CJ. Conjunctivitis in birds. Vet Clin N Am Exotic Anim Pract 2002;5:287–399.

28. Pocknell AM, Miller BJ, Neufeld JL, Grahn BH. Conjunctival mycobacteriosis in two emus (*Dromaius novaehollandiae*). Vet Pathol 1996;33:346–348.

29. Wolf ED, Amass K, Olsen J. Survey of conjunctival flora in the eye of clinically normal, captive exotic birds. J Am Vet Med Assoc 1983;183:1232–1233.

30. Zenoble RD, Griffith RW, Clubb SL. Survey of bacteriologic flora of conjunctiva and cornea in healthy psittacine birds. Am J Vet Res 1983;44:1966–1967.

31. Crispin SM, Barnett KC. Ocular candidiasis in ornamental ducks. Avian Pathol 1978;7:49–59.

32. Surman PG, Schultz DJ, Tham VL. Keratoconjunctivitis and chlamydiosis in cage birds. Aust Vet J 1974;50:356–362.

33. Schwabe CW. Studies on *Oxyspirura mansoni*, the tropical eyeworm of poultry. III. Preliminary observations on eyeworm pathogenicity. Am J Vet Res 1950;11:286–290.

34. Brooks DE, Greiner EC, Walsh MT. Conjunctivitis caused by *Thelazia* sp in a Senegal parrot. J Am Vet Med Assoc 183:1305–1306.

35. Greve JH, Harrison GJ. Conjunctivitis caused by eye flukes in captive-reared ostriches. J Am Vet Med Assoc 1980;77:909–910.

36. Korbel R, Schäffer EH. The occurrence of conjunctivitis of unknown etiology in budgerigars (*Melopsittacus undulatus*, Shaw 1805). Tierarztl Prax 1991;19:659–663.

37. Karpinski LG, SL Clubb. Post pox ocular problems in Blue-fronted Amazons and Blue-headed Pionus Parrots. Proceedings of AAV Annual Conference, 1985.

38. Karpinski LG, SL Clubb. An outbreak of avian pox in imported mynahs. Proceedings of AAV Annual Conference, 1986.

39. Bonous DI, Schaeffer DO, Roy A. Coagulase-negtaive *Staphylococcus* sp. septicaemia in a lovebird. J Am Vet Med Assoc 1989;195:1120–1121.

40. van den Brand JM, Manvell R, Paul G, Kik MJ, Dorrestein GM. Reovirus infections associated with high mortality in psittaciformes in The Netherlands. Avian Pathol 2007;36:293–299.

41. Clubb SL, Karpinski LG. Aging in macaws. J Ass Avian Vet 1993;7:31–33.

42. Carter RT, Murphy CJ, Stuhr CM, Diehl KA. Bilateral phacoemulsification and intraocular lens implantation in a great horned owl. J Am Vet Med Assoc 2007;230:559–561.

43. Van Niekerk WH, Petrick SW. Unilateral lentectomy in a black-shouldered kite. J S Afr Vet Assoc 1990;61:124–125.

44. Brooks DE, Murphy CJ, Quesenberry KE, Walsh MT. Surgical correction of a luxated cataractous lens in a barred owl. J Am Vet Med Assoc 1983;183:1298–1299.

45. Williams DL, Gonzalez Villavincencio CM, Wilson S. Chronic ocular lesions in tawny owls (*Strix aluco*) injured by road traffic. Vet Rec 2006;159:148–153.

46. Bayon A, Almela RM, Talavera J. Avian ophthalmology. Eur J Comp Anim Pract 2007;17:253–265.

47. Moore PA, Munnell JF, Martin CL, Prasse KW, Carmichael KP. Photoreceptor cell dysplasia in two Tippler pigeons. Vet Ophthalmol 2004;7:197–203.

48. Dukes TW, Fox GA. Blindness associated with retinal dysplasia in a prairie falcon, *Falco mexicanus*. J Wildl Dis 1983;19:66–69.

49. Montiani-Ferreira F, Li T, Kiupel M, Howland H, Hocking P, Curtis R, Petersen-Jones S. Clinical features of the retinopathy, globe enlarged (rge) chick phenotype. Vision Res 2003;43: 2009–2018.

50. Montiani-Ferreira F, Fischer A, Cernuda-Cernuda R, Kiupel M, DeGrip WJ, Sherry D, Cho SS, Shaw GC, Evans MG, Hocking PM, Petersen-Jones SM. Detailed histopathologic characterization of the retinopathy, globe enlarged (rge) chick phenotype. Mol Vis 2005;11: 11–27.

51. Montiani-Ferreira F, Shaw GC, Geller AM, Petersen-Jones SM. Electroretinographic features of the retinopathy, globe enlarged (rge) chick phenotype. Mol Vis 2007;13:553–565.

52. Tudor DC, Yard C. Retinal atrophy in a parakeet. Vet Med Small Anim Clin 1978;73:1456.

53. Williams SM, Fulton RM, Render JA, Mansfield L, Bouldin M. Ocular and encephalic toxoplasmosis in canaries. Avian Dis 2001;45:262–267.
54. Vickers MC, Hartley WJ, Mason RW, Dubey JP, Schollam L. (1992) Blindness associated with toxoplasmosis in canaries. J Am Vet Med Assoc 1992;200:1723–1725.
55. Williams DL, Cooper JE. Horner's syndrome in an African spotted eagle owl (*Bubo africanus*). Vet Rec 1994;134:64–66.
56. Gancz AY, Lee S, Higginson G, Danylyk I, Smith DA, Taylor M. Horner's syndrome in an eastern screech owl (*Megascops asio*). Vet Rec 2006;159:320–322.
57. Canton DD, Murphy CJ, Buyukmihci NC, Schulz T. Pupilloplasty in a great horned owl with pupillary occlusion and cataracts. J Am Vet Med Assoc 1992;201:1087–1090.
58. Gionfriddo JR, Powell CC. Primary closure of the corneas of two great horned owls after resection of nonhealing ulcers. Vet Ophthalmol 2006;9:251–254.
59. Andrew SE, Clippinger TL, Brooks DE, Helmick KE. Penetrating keratoplasty for treatment of corneal protrusion in a great horned owl (*Bubo virginianus*). Vet Ophthalmol 2002;5: 201–205.
60. Murphy CJ, Brooks DE, Kern TJ, Quesenberry KE, Riis RC. Enucleation in birds of prey. J Am Vet Med Assoc 1983;183:1234–1237.
61. Christen C, Richter M, Fischer I, Eule C, Spiess B, Hatt JM. Unilateral evisceration of an eye following cornea and lens perforation in a sulfur-crested cockatoo (*Cacatua galerita*). Schweiz Arch Tierheilkd 2006;148:615–619.
62. Implantation of an intraocular silicone prosthesis in a great horned owl (*Bubo virginianus*). J Avian Med Surg 1999;13:98–103.
63. Hegemann A, Hegemann ED, Krone O. Successful rehabilitation and release with a subsequent brood of a one-eyed eagle owl (*Bubo bubo*). Berl Munch Tierarztl Wochenschr 2007; 120:183–188.

# Chapter 10

# The reptile eye

## Introduction

Any review of reptile ophthalmology, must refer back to a key work on the subject, that of Millichamp, Jacobson and Wolf [1], which even though it is now over 25 years old, still provides much useful information. Other overviews include that of Lawton, whose chapter in the second edition of Mader's *Reptile Medicine and Surgery* [2], added to my contribution to the smaller first edition [3]. Here I will aim to bring new data to the field as well as covering that already known. We will concentrate on diseases of reptiles kept as pets or in zoological collections but will include some conditions seen in wild reptiles in order to compare and contrast with what may be encountered in captive reptiles. These animals, perhaps in contradistinction to the mammals and birds already covered, are still very much wild animals in captivity, and thus diseases seen in their counterparts free in the wild, are perhaps of more relevance than in captive wild mammals or birds.

## Anatomy and physiology of the reptilian eye

The key monograph on reptile ocular anatomy is Underwood's masterful chapter in the second volume of Gans and Parsons' *Biology of the Reptilia* [4]. Gordon Lynn Walls in his classic text [5] and Sir Stewart Duke Elder in his *The Eye in Evolution* [6] both also contribute valuably to the literature on the reptile eye, although the age of these publications means they do not include more modern research.

The eyes of lizards, snakes, crocodilians and chelonia are surprisingly different, these variations giving considerable insight into both the diversity of their evolutionary origins and their current residence in different ecological niches. As Underwood notes in his introduction 'The eye shows how species have modified their basic equipment to current conditions and evolutionary opportunities. Study of the eye may contribute to reconstruction of a group's phylogeny' [4]. Following Underwood we will start by describing the eye and adnexa of a typical diurnal lizard.

The large orbits contain the extraocular muscles, the large Harderian gland which curls around the globe at its posterior aspect, the lacrimal gland and an orbital sinus which

*Ophthalmology of Exotic Pets*, First Edition. David L. Williams.
© 2012 David Williams. Published 2012 by Blackwell Publishing Ltd.

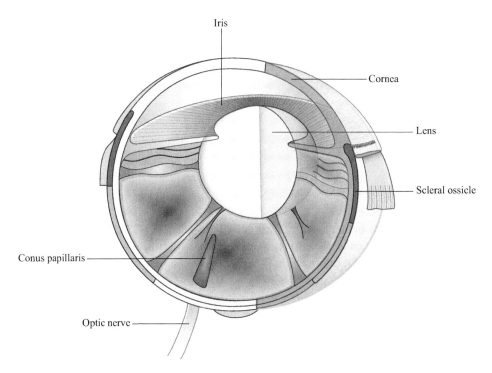

**Figure 10.1**   Line diagram of lizard eye.

connects to the internal jugular vein via the vena cerebralis, clearly an important fact to be borne in mind when considering enucleation. The orbits meet medially with only a cartilaginous septum between them, meaning that an abscess in one orbit could readily cross to the fellow orbit, although in practice this is rarely if ever seen. The eyelids are unequal with the upper eyelid, although containing smooth muscle, being relatively immobile. The eye opens predominantly through downward movement of the lower eyelid which contains a large cartilaginous plate. In several families of lizard and in all snakes the eyelids are fused to form a transparent spectacle, the biology and diseases of which will be discussed further below. In those lizards with eyelids, the nictitating membrane, a fold of conjunctiva, contains vertical crescents of cartilage attached to a tendon which links them to the retrobulbar bursalis muscle. Thus while conjunctival flaps can be fashioned in a similar manner to those in cats and dogs, the tension on them from the action of this bursalis muscle often renders them of use for only a short time before the suture tears through. A tarsorraphy may be of more benefit.

The globe of the lizard eye (Figure 10.1) can be divided into an anterior corneal and a posterior orbital segment. The cornea has a thin stroma but a relatively thick Bowman's layer covered by a thin corneal epithelium. The iridocorneal angle is poorly developed compared with that of higher vertebrates. Overlapping scleral ossicles, around 10–14 in lizards, are found in the sclera immediately behind the limbus overlying the ciliary body which, as Underwood puts it, embraces the equator of the lens. Crampton's muscle and Brucke's muscle lie between the ciliary body and the sclera with actions in accommodation, since contraction of Crampton's muscle draws the ciliary body anteriorly pressing it against the lens and shortening its focal length. This allows not only changes in the lens sphericity but also enhancement of the curvature of the cornea. The lens is fairly soft with an epithelium which thickens markedly at the lens equator forming the *Ringwulst* which brings the lens into contact with the ciliary body. Nocturnal lizards such as the spectacled geckos have very large corneas with an almost spherical lens and a pupil which is hexagonal when dilated, allowing a much larger pupil diameter than that of a circular pupil, and closes to a slit on miosis. Diurnal lizards are more likely to have a simple round pupil. Not only does iris anatomy differ between lizards with such different lifestyles. The depth of the globe along its optical axis is significantly less in noctural lizards, allowing much greater irradiance of the viewed image on the retina in the nocturnal reptile species [7]. The differences in visually orientated behaviour between nocturnal and diurnal lizards is also manifest in their photoreceptor populations. All diurnal lizards have retinas populated solely by cones, both single and double, with oil droplets giving them specific responses to particular light wavelengths. Nocturnal species within this group, such as the nocturnal geckos, have cones which have developed morphological features of rods but still contain and use cone photopigments in their visual transduction pathway.

As noted above and discussed further below, the eyes of all snakes are covered by a spectacle formed from fused transparent eyelids. The ophidian eye (Figure 10.2) is sufficiently different from that of other reptile groups for Walls to conclude that it developed

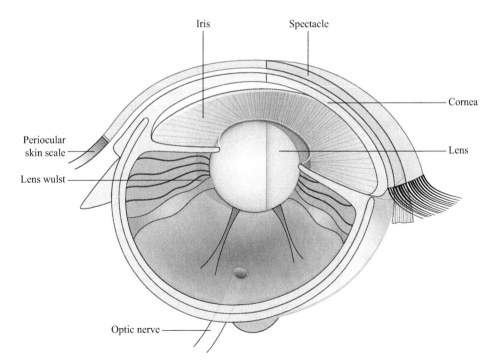

**Figure 10.2**   Line diagram of snake eye.

a second time from an almost vestigial eye which had degenerated during an evolutionary period spent underground. Regarding the difference between the snake eye and that of other reptiles, Underwood goes so far as to suggest that 'there is nothing about [the snake eye] to suggest that its owner is a reptile, let alone one related to lizards' [8]. The ophidian orbit has only the Harderian gland, which secretes a seromucous fluid between the spectacle and the cornea [9] rather than also having a lacrimal gland producing a less viscous fluid as do all other reptiles. Snakes do not have scleral ossicles but have an entirely fibrous sclera with a cartilaginous cup posteriorly. The cornea, not needing to have a protective function since that is taken over by the spectacle, is thin with an epithelium only of a very few cell layers. Snakes accommodate with changes in lens deformation but more importantly also by forward movement of the lens. The relative importance of these two mechanisms is unclear, and in his significant cross-species review Ott argues that further research is needed and that at present any definitive statements on ophidian accommodation should be treated with caution [10].

The chelonian eye varies markedly between species, predominantly because of the different ecological niches they inhabit. The amphibious terrapin *Emys*, for instance, has a relatively convex cornea and a thick lens with a thin annular pad [11]. To have appropriate refraction above and below the water such aquatic chelonia use their iris to squeeze the anterior face of the lens, dramatically increasing its curvature. In terrestrial *Testudo* species the lens is less spherical, since in its terrestrial environment the cornea plays an active part in light refraction but the small ocular size of many of these species still means that the lens cannot be as ovoid as that of larger mammals.

The eyelids are positioned so that the lateral canthus is higher than the medial. While this means that an aquatic terrapin or turtle rising to the surface has its palpebral aperture parallel to the water surface, it is not clear why terrestrial species maintain this anatomical peculiarity. The nictitating membrane is pronounced, being withdrawn by the pyramidalis muscle. The lacrimal and Harderian glands are large in most chelonia compared to other reptiles and especially so in marine species and those inhabiting brackish water since they have been shown to excrete salt [12]. Photoreceptors of chelonia comprise a predominant cone population with single and double cones with oil droplets; while some suggest the chelonian retina is devoid of rods, Walls describes rods in several species [5].

## Biology of the reptilian spectacle

As we noted in the introduction to this volume, a key feature of exotic animal ophthalmology as with any area of exotic animal medicine, is knowing when extrapolation from what one already knows of more conventional pet anatomy, physiology and disease is appropriate and where one needs new information concerning differences between the species being investigated and those with which one is more familiar.

This is nowhere more true than in the case of the snake spectacle. Here, assuming that we can extrapolate from what is already known in the cat or dog will result in incorrect diagnoses and potentially damaging treatments. All snakes, and a reasonable proportion of lizards, have a transparent covering over the cornea, presumably for protection. This is the spectacle or, as it used to be termed by the biologists who first investigated it, the 'brille'.

The spectacle is formed from fusion of the eyelids and thus forms a closed space in which the tears form, circulate and are drained through the nasolacrimal duct. This marked difference from the anatomy of the open ocular surface in all other animals has a substantial influence on both the normal anatomy and physiology of the area and the disease states experienced in the eye where the spectacle is present. As the spectacle is formed from skin structures it has characteristics of the skin scales including blood vessels, as beautifully shown by Dr A Mead in his study (Figure 10.3) [13]. The spectacle is shed with the rest of the skin and during this period of shedding it becomes oedematous and opaque as quite a normal phase in growth of the animal (Figure 10.4). Obstruction of the nasolacrimal duct in any other animal would result in epiphora, that is to say tear overflow. In reptiles with a spectacle such a pathology leads to swelling of the spectacle in what is known as bullous spectaculopathy. We will see further below other diseases specific to reptiles with spectacles and discuss their management as well as essential husbandry principles if diseases of the spectacle are to be avoided.

The evolution of the spectacle is a somewhat controversial area of debate. Most pale-ontologists accept that snakes evolved from terrestrial squamates although the fossil

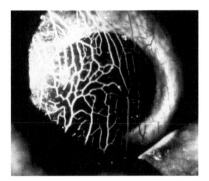

**Figure 10.3**  A vascular cast of the vessels in the normal snake spectacle. (Courtesy of Dr A Mead.)

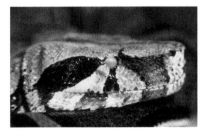

**Figure 10.4**  Opacity of the snake spectacle during ecdysis. (Reproduced with permission from Professor Elliott Jacobson.)

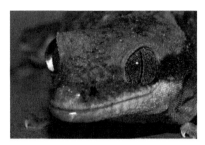

**Figure 10.5**   A normal Sarasin's giant gecko (*Rhacodactylus sarasinorum*) showing the extent of the subspectacular space although total internal reflection may exaggerate the depth between cornea and spectacle. (Reproduced with permission from Dr Stephen Barten.)

record of early snakes is not as complete as we might wish it to be. Snake skeletons are generally small and fragile and as such good fossilised examples are rare. Having said that specimens from 150 million years ago have been identified as early snakes but with skeletal structures eminently lizard-like, these mostly found in South America. Such burrowing lizards could quite feasibly have developed fused eyelids to protect the cornea during burrowing at the same time as experiencing the loss of external ears and overt limbs. The pythons and boas of today, generally held to be more primitive groups of snakes, still have vestigial hind limbs demonstrating how feasible such an evolutionary development could be.

Another group suggest that prototypic snakes developed form monosaurs, extinct aquatic reptiles of the Cretaceous period. If this were the case the spectacle developed to combat environmental threats quite different from the adbrasions of the subterrestrial world, namely the loss of water though the cornea by osmosis when the animal was living in an salty aquatic environment. On this theory the snakes recolonised the land in the late Cretaceous period. Cladistic studies comparing snakes with monosaurs are suggested to support such a hypothesis as does the finding of snake fossil remains in marine sediments from the late Cretaceous period.

The presence of a spectacle in the geckos (Figure 10.5) is difficult to explain using either of these theories of origins. It may be that convergent evolution has resulted in eyelid fusion in these lizards with their large protuberant eyes where ocular surface protection is all important.

## What do reptiles see?

Nobody would attempt to ask or answer such a broad question as 'what do mammals see?', realizing that this group of animals covers everything from rats to cats, not forgetting bats! Yet somehow we expect to be able to cover what reptiles see in a paragraph or two. But reptiles range from crocodilians, with dorsally placed eyes, to boa constrictors and pythons with their eyes fully lateralised. Reptiles range from nocturnal species

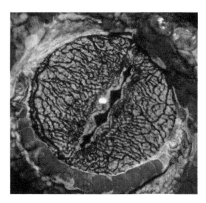

**Figure 10.6**  The polchorate (many pupilled) iris of the Tockay gecko.

such as the leopard gecko to diurnal animals like inland bearded dragons with obvious differences in vision and its importance in behaviour. The nocturnal geckos such as the leopard gecko, somewhat surprisingly, have a rodless retina with nocturnal colour vision, since they have evolved from cone-dominated diurnal lizards [14]. Diurnal snakes such as the garter snake, understandably have a cone-rich retina [15], while those that hunt nocturnally are more rod-dominated [16]. Such differences in activity in different light levels are reflected throughout the eye and not just in the retina; snakes whose habits are diurnal have round pupils while nocturnal snakes have slit pupils allowing a wider range of light entry [17].

What then of their field of vision? Again many snakes have laterally placed eyes giving an almost panoramic field of vision while the diurnal geckos have forward facing eyes with a substantial field of binocular vision. It has to be said, however, that no researcher has studied the extent of visual fields in reptiles in the same way that Graham Martin has for their avian counterparts (see page xx). We know from studies of unilaterally anophthalmic snakes that vision with both eyes, even if this may not involve a truly stereo binocular field, is important in prey location [18]. An interesting feature of certain reptiles with regard to prey location is the multiple pupils of reptiles such as the Tockay gecko (Figure 10.6). This anatomy yields a refractive arrangement whereby only objects at the focal distance of the lens appear as one in-focus image on the retina. In this manner these animals are able to determine the distance of a prey item prior to capture [19].

Many reptiles have two other sensory modalities for detecting electromagnetic radiation. The first detects light, and with an organ analogous to the lateral eyes; the parietal eye homolous with the pineal gland of higher vertebrates. In lower vertebrates such as the lizards, the parietal eye is histologically similar to the conventional eyes (Figure 10.7). These mid-brain structures are overlain by a dorsal foramen in the skull, the pineal foramen, and a translucent skin scale which in the tuatara *Sphenodon punctatus* has corneal-like focusing power. The parietal eye plays a central role in diurnal and seasonal

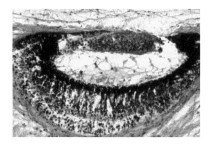

**Figure 10.7**   Parietal eye of *Lacerta sicula*, the wall lizard.

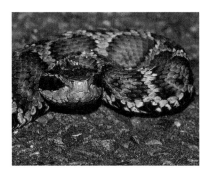

**Figure 10.8**   Pit organs.

physiological and behavioural cycles through light detection and a more hardwired manner than the effects of the pineal gland in higher vertebrates.

Secondly a number of reptiles, most specifically snakes such as the crotaline pit vipers but also boids, use infrared detection in predation. In boids, such as the Burmese python, nerves from the infrared end-organs located deep within invaginations between labial scales (Figure 10.8) project from the trigeminal ganglion to the lateral descending nucleus of the trigeminal tract (LTTD), a brainstem nucleus found only in snakes with infrared detection and apparently devoted to processing such information. In the crotaline pit vipers a single pit organ contains an infrared-sensitive membrane from whence the nerves proceed to the LTTD and thus on to the nucleus reticularis caloris and lateral tegmental nucleus. These nerve flows are clearly very different from that of cranial nerve II, the optic nerve, where the majority of impulses flow to the contralateral tectum. However both imaging systems eventually project to the tectum where they converge to form overlying spatial maps in rather the same way that barn owls coordinate their visual and auditory tectal spatial maps. Research evaluating prey capture has shown that deprivation of either sight or infrared detection did not alter rattlesnakes' strike behaviour or ability to catch prey [20], while obliteration of both systems led to greater strike latency, fewer strikes and less accurate contact with prey [21,22]. A congenitally blind rattlesnake, however, showed no difference in behaviour than a normally sighted sibling [23].

# Diseases of the reptile eye

## *Hypovitaminosis A in chelonians*

### *Clinical signs*

Signs of hypovitaminosis A can range from mild eyelid oedema through to much more severe eyelid swelling with hyperaemic chemotic conjunctiva enlarged to the extent that the lids are closed with no globe visible and the animal rendered blind (Figure 10.9). It is important to note that vitamin A deficiency in chelonia may also be involved in combination with infectious or traumatic factors in ocular disease (Figure 10.10). Even at the early stages of the disease respiratory pathology may also be evident. While the clinical picture may be considered pathognomonic and further diagnostic tests rendered superfluous, biopsy of the conjunctiva can show disintegrating epithelial cells,

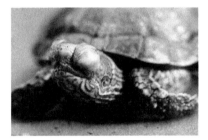

**Figure 10.9** Dr Edward Elkan's first photograph of a terrapin with hypovitaminosis A. (Reproduced with permission from the Edward Elkan Collection of Lower Vertebrate Pathology and the Journal of Zoo and Wildlife Medicine.)

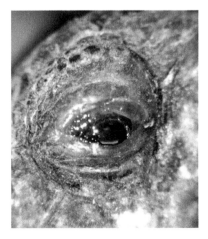

**Figure 10.10** A Greek spur-thighed tortoise *Testudo graeca* with infectious blepharitis after hibernation. Note that vitamin A deficiency may also be a contributory factor here.

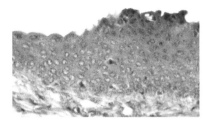

**Figure 10.11**   Histopathology of hypovitaminosis A. (Reproduced with permission from the Edward Elkan Collection of Lower Vertebrate Pathology and the Journal of Zoo and Wildlife Medicine.)

hyperkeratinised epithelium and keratin pearls with granulocyte infiltration as a feature occurring secondary to infection. Since the freshwater aquatic chelonia thus affected are sight-feeders, these blinding ocular changes further exacerbate the nutritional deficiency at their heart.

Dermal signs of the vitamin A deficiency on the eyelids may also be seen later in the disease and dermal hyperkeratosis of the eyelids has been reported in juvenile sea turtles [24].

### Aetiopathogenesis

It was nearly 50 years ago that Dr Edward Elkan and Dr Peer Zwart independently identified hypovitaminosis as the cause of the conjunctival changes seen in aquatic chelonia with poor nutritional status, publishing their findings together in 1967 [25]. Their histopathological studies demonstrated epithelial changes in conjunctiva and orbital glands which were characteristic of low vitamin A levels (Figure 10.11). Hypovitaminosis A is particularly obvious in terrapins because of the large proportion of the orbit occupied by the lacrimal and Harderian glands. Lizards generally have a ventromedial Harderian gland and a dorsotemporal lacrimal gland but these are considerably smaller than in the freshwater aquatic chelonia. Geckos, chameleons and snakes have only a well developed Harderian gland, but even this does not rival the size of the chelonian orbital glands. The desquamated hyperkeratinised epithelium swells the conjunctiva and fills the orbit.

### Clinical management

As noted above the clinical signs of vitamin A deficiency in freshwater aquatic chelonia are essentially pathognomonic rendering biopsy unnecessary, but cytology can be useful not only to confirm the diagnosis but to allow evaluation of inflammation and infection, common secondary features of the disease. Should impression cytology reveal numerous heterophils or bacteria, topical and perhaps even systemic antibiosis with a fluoroquinolone such as enrofloxacin or ciprofloxacin may be necessary.

The key feature of management of the condition is, however, restoration of a correct level of vitamin A. This can be by weekly intramuscular injection of water-soluble vitamin A. Some argue that this can all too commonly result in hypervitaminosis A, but oral dosing can be fruitless, since the intestinal epithelium can be similarly dystrophic, rendering absorption of dietary vitamin A difficult if not impossible. Having said that it is important to be aware of the signs of hypervitaminosis A, those of skin sloughing and blister formation.

## Periocular lesions – infection and inflammation

### Clinical signs

Periocular adnexal lesions in reptiles may involve lid swelling (Figure 10.12), ocular discharge and conjunctival hyperaemia. It is important to note the variations present in normal eyes between species. Some varanid monitor lizards, for example, have a vivid red episclera which is quite within normal limits while in another species this would be a sign of ocular inflammation.

### Aetiopathogenesis

The most common cause of eyelid pathology in reptiles is hypovitaminosis A as discussed above. Nevertheless blepharitis and conjunctivitis have been noted with other causes; infection either local or systemic, this being particularly important as conjunctivitis may occur as a sequel to septicaemia. We will however start with localized causes of adnexal lesions. Trauma can lead to significant adnexal pathology either directly (Figure 10.13) or with substrate occluding the palpebral aperture (see Figure 10.16).

Viral disease may manifest as adnexal pathology; caiman pox has been reported with focal raised white or cream-coloured papules (Figure 10.14) [26]. These lesions may occur anywhere on the skin but are perhaps most commonly seen on the delicate skin of the eyelid.

Herpesvirus infection has been reported associated with proliferative and often ulcerative skin lesions in sea turtles [27] as well as with tracheitis and conjunctivitis in the same species and periocular neoplasms (Figure 10.15) [28]. Research has demonstrated association of two very similar herpesviruses in green sea turtles (*Chelonia mydas*) and loggerhead turtle (*Caretta caretta)* in Florida. Secondary bacterial infection often occurs in association with these lesions.

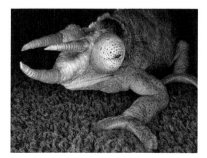

**Figure 10.12**   Rhinoceros iguana with periocular swelling.

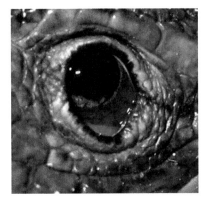

**Figure 10.13**   Ectropion following deflation of a periorbital cyst in a water dragon.

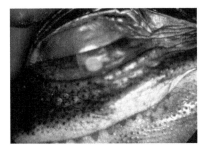

**Figure 10.14**   Caiman pox lesion in eyelid of caiman. (Reproduced with permission from Professor Elliott Jacobson.)

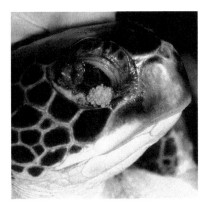

**Figure 10.15**   Herpes-virus-associated fibropapilloma in *Chelonia mydas*. (Reproduced with permission from Professor Elliott Jacobson.)

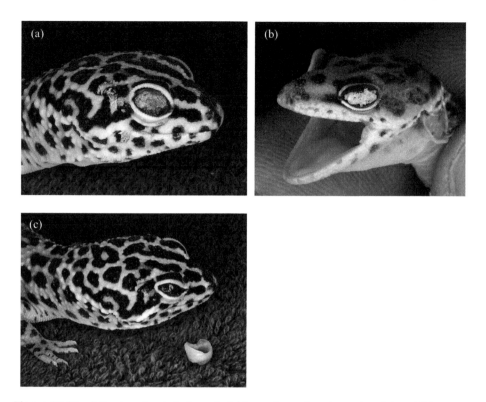

**Figure 10.16** Adhesion of substrate material to ocular surface in geckos (a) and (b), requiring careful removal with microsurgical forceps (c).

## Conjunctivitis

### Clinical signs

Conjunctivitis in reptiles is most often associated with blepharitis, with eyelid swelling and sometimes chemosis, sometimes with a mucoid discharge but often with the eyelids being sealed shut with a dry caseous discharge (Figure 10.16).

### Aetiopathogenesis

Adnexal lesions with infectious origins more likely to be seen in captive pet reptiles are those associated with bacterial disease and can be important signs that septicaemia is occurring, although they may be localized to the eye alone. Periocular *Aeromonas* infections, for example, were noted to cause conjunctivitis and blepharitis in a colony of lacertid lizards [29], while *Pseudomonas* was isolated from a group of anoles with conjunctivitis and blepharitis. The lacertid lizards first developed a clear fluid discharge, difficult to detect initially, which eventually led to the lids sealing closed with associated visual impairment and anorexia. Death occurred within a week of the lids sealing closed. Histopathology revealed a mucoprulent ocular discharge and a prevalent growth of

*Aeromonas liquifaciens.* Treatment in the first group with oral oxytetracycline and topical ocular bathing was successful while the anoles responded well to topical gentamicin. Vivarium hygiene was improved and ventilation increased with some effect. The meal-worms comprising the majority of the diet were thought to be a potential source of infection, but changing their source had no effect on the infection.

*Chlamydophila* is generally considered a conjunctival pathogen in birds more than in reptiles, but exudative conjunctivitis has been reported associated with *Chlamydia* in hatchling and juvenile crocodiles in a farm in New Guinea [30]. While this may be thought to have little relevance to pet reptiles, the problem in this situation was one introduced by the unquarantined introduction of wild-caught animals into the farm. Such a report confirms the importance of ensuring strict biosecurity when introducing new individuals into any group of captive animals.

Other causes of conjunctivitis can include irritation from physical causes, such as small pieces of vermiculite used as a substrate, through to chemical agents, such as organo-chlorine pesticides reported to be associated with conjunctivitis, belpharitis and ocular discharge in eastern box turtles [31]; such agencies are less likely to be the cause than systemic infection, in this author's experience.

### Clinical management

In all these cases noted above bacteriological investigation was central to a correct diagnosis as was a thorough ophthalmogical examination. Note however that the health of the whole animal must also be evaluated since many of these ocular signs are harbingers of systemic infection. Topical and systemic antibiotics should be prescribed but a key first step is opening the sealed palpebral aperture, seen in many cases, with warm water compresses.

## Periocular masses

### Clinical signs

Periocular masses in reptiles present as a firm swelling gradually increasing in size (Figure 10.17 and Figure 10.18), with signs of secondary trauma caused by their size and the blindness they cause.

### Aetiopathogenesis

The vast majority of these are inflammatory lesions secondary to Gram-negative bacterial or fungal infection. In reptiles these inflammatory lesions are for the most part granulo-matous in nature and not the fluid-filled mass of, say, a cat-bite abscess. They can thus be very difficult to differentiate from neoplasms which can also be seen in this area. Indeed adnexal mass lesions may be inflammatory, infectious and neoplastic concurrently, as Abou-Madi and Kern show in their report of a squamous cell carcinoma together with abscessation with *Pseudomonas aeruginosa* [32]. Others are purely infectious, as in the periorbital abscess in a chameleon reported by Schumacher and colleagues [33].

Other causes of adnexal pathology include parasitic infestations with surgical exploration of one in a chameleon revealing microfilaria of the fillaroid genus (in that case

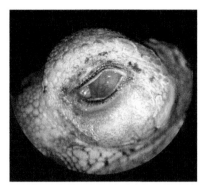

**Figure 10.17**   Periocular abscess in an iguana.

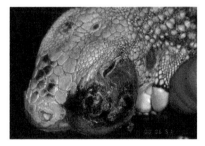

**Figure 10.18**   Periocular abscess in an iguana.

*Foleyella*, a relatively common parasite in chameleons). Cystic structures associated with the nasolacrimal system can also occur with dacryops, an acquired lacrimal cyst reported in a terrapin resulting in periocular swelling together with exophthalmos [34]; another report demonstrated a vascular anomaly, an orbital varies, as a cause of exophthalmos and periocular swelling [35].

As noted earlier, the heterophilic inflammatory cell infiltrate in reptiles followed by macrophages, leads to a granulomatous reponse with formation of giant cells somewhat similar to those in the caseous lesions seen in mycobacterial disease in man. The abscesses seen in reptiles are thus mostly solid at their core rather than fluid pus-filled as with neutrophil-dominated abscesses in mammals [36].

## Clinical management

Management of a periocular mass must clearly be dictated by the specific diagnosis reached, but in most cases surgical exploration and resection will be important in both reaching a diagnosis and dealing with the lesion itself. Whether purely infectious, neoplastic, or fibrous reactive lesion, surgical removal is the key to resolution of the lesion. Note however that the relatively thin skin of the ocular adnexa in reptiles means that a mass in this area readily distorts the eyelid margins as seen in Figure 10.15, rendering vision problematic in many cases. Reconstructive surgery may well be required to bring the palpebral aperture in apposition with the globe.

### Dacryocystitis

#### Clinical signs

Inflammation of the nasolacrimal duct can be seen in several reptiles, even those in which, according to the anatomy books, no nasolacrimal duct exists! Thus, while some text books report that chelonia do not have a nasolacrimal duct, dacryocystitis has been reported in these species, with discharge and bubble formation at the medial canthus. Animals with epiphora – tear overflow – or a purulent ocular discharge particularly from the medial canthus should be investigated for dacryocystitis with slit lamp biomicrscopy and placement of a drop of fluorescein dye in the eye to assess appearance of the dye at the external nares.

#### Management

Topical and systemic antibiotics together with regular flushing, if possible, might be suggested.

### Opacity of the spectacle

The normally clear spectacle may become opaque for one of several reasons. The most common is that before ecdysis, as noted above, the spectacle becomes opaque, as fluid increases to separate the old spectacle from the newly formed tissue underneath (Figure 10.19). The whole skin becomes dull for the same reason and this is a normal appearance at the time of ecdysis. Most commonly just before shedding occurs the spectacle clears, comfirming that this is part of the snake's normal growth. Should retention of the spectacle occur some opacity may occur, but this is not the dense white of the shedding

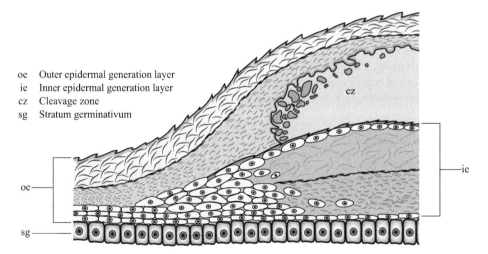

oe   Outer epidermal generation layer
ie   Inner epidermal generation layer
cz   Cleavage zone
sg   Stratum germinativum

**Figure 10.19**   Histological changes in snake skin as ecdysis occurs.

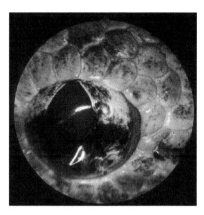

**Figure 10.20**   Indentation of the spectacle after trauma.

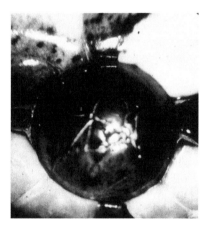

**Figure 10.21**   Pigmentation of the superficial layers of an old spectacle.

spectacle, rather a dull lustreless appearance. This condition is covered further below. Another cause of opacity in the spectacle can be trauma. Given that the whole point of the spectacle is to protect the underlying cornea, continued mild trauma can lead to scratches on the spectacle, indentation of the surface (Figure 10.20) or more severe pigmentation (Figure 10.21). Such opacification is not of concern, however, since the new spectacle revealed after shedding will be clear and transparent. Bullous spectaculopathy (see below), where a fluid accumulation distends the spectacle, can also lead to opacification possibly from trauma, although in many cases the distended spectacle is clear.

## Retained spectacle

### Clinical signs

Retention of previously unshed spectacles is manifest as a raised plaque of retained tissue, often opaque, in the ocular area and often too with a 'frill' of scale remains around

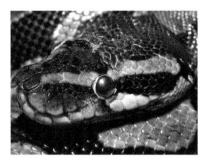

**Figure 10.22**   Retained spectacle in a *Python regius*. (Reproduced with permission from Dr Stephen Barten.)

the edge of the spectacle (Figure 10.22). It is often the case that these retained 'eyecaps' are multiple. Differential diagnoses include opacity of the spectacle through infection or trauma, bullous spectaculopathy (see below) or a subspectacular abscess. Another, but much less common differential diagnosis would be one of a neoplastic process such as a keratoacanthoma [37]. The multiple nature of these retained layers of skin is normally obvious on close examination.

### Aetiopathogenesis

Spectacle retention is often seen as part of a more generalissed dysecdysis where skin shedding is not complete (Figure 10.22). This may be associated with generalised poor health but more often than not the underlying problem is a husbandry deficit and particularly too low a humidity. This is understandable given that the separation of newly regenerated and old epithelium in the skin scales – and also the spectacle – relies on the generation of a fluid-filled delineation between the two layers. Thus a snake kept in too low a humidity is likely to suffer dysecdysis with attendant spectacle retention. Another aetiopathogenic factor of a number of cases is infestation with the snake mite *Ophionyssus natricis*. This parasite itself undergoes several moults as it reaches adulthood. Between each of these it takes a blood meal to increase its body size and the easiest place to take such a meal is the space between the spectacle and the first periocular skin scale. Multiple punctures here cause inflammation and lead to spectacle retention. The dark deposits around the spectacles in Figure 10.23 are the mites (Figure 10.24) and the haemorrhagic remains of their multiple blood meals.

### Clinical management

The key point to note in managing a case of retained spectacle is that no attempt should be made to remove the retained tissue by force, using a pair of forceps. This will all too often result in removal of the entire spectacle with a resultant severe keratitis as shown in Figure 10.25. We have noted that low humidity is critical in many cases of retained spectacles. Increasing the humidity at the time of next ecdysis may be sufficient to promote a full shed with removal of the retained spectacles. If this is not the case use of

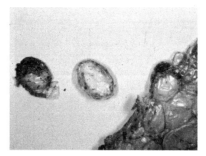

**Figure 10.23** Retained spectacles seen after a successful shed. Note the black debris around the spectacle, indicative of *Ophionyssus* infestation, an important causative factor in spectacle retention. (Reproduced with permission from Dr Stephen Barten.)

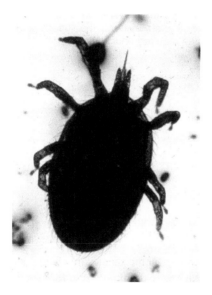

**Figure 10.24** The snake mite *Ophionyssus natricis.* (Reproduced with permission from Dr Stephen Barten.)

damp cotton paper in the vivarium against which the snake can rub itself, or soaked cotton wool abraded against the retained spectacles can affect removal of the abnormal tissue. A recalcitrant mass of spectacles can be removed with forceps if no other less severe technique has a beneficial effect, but such a technique is best achieved with the snake under a general anaesthetic and using an operating microscope to ensure that the true spectacle and underlying eye are not damaged.

### Prophylaxis

Keeping the snake in an appropriate humidity, especially around the time of shedding, is vitally important if dysecdysis and spectacle retention are to be avoided. The correct

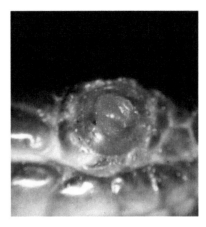

**Figure 10.25**   Severe keratitis after the removal of the entire spectacle in a corn snake with retained spectacles in an attempt to remove only the superficial retained tissue. Management of this catastrophe required enucleation.

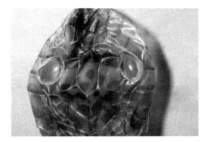

**Figure 10.26**   Shed skin or exuvium with both spectacles correctly shed.

level will clearly differ depending on the species involved – a desert dwelling snake will require a lower humidity than one residing in a rain forest, although even here it should be noted that the microclimate inhabited by the animal may be considerably more humid than one would expect in a desert habitat. Providing a damp area within the vivarium is worthwhile and wetted paper added to the vivarium at the time of moulting is valuable, especially in an animal which has previously been affected by spectacle retention.

Owners with snakes thus affected should be encouraged to check at each shed that the exuvium (the shed skin) includes both shed spectacles (Figure 10.26) to ensure that a set of retained spectacles does not build up and that preventative measures can be taken if dysecdysis occurs.

### Bullous spectaculopathy

#### Clinical signs

Obstruction of the nasolacrimal ducts in snakes leads to a build up of tear fluid under the spectacle with resultant marked enlargement of the spectacle. The resulting appear-

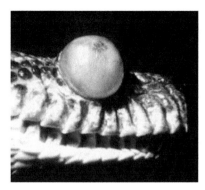

**Figure 10.27**  Protuberant opaque spectacle in bullous spectaculopathy. (Reproduced with permission from Dr Fredric Frye. Originally printed in *Biological and Surgical Aspects of Captive Reptile Husbandry*, 2nd Ed., 1991, Krieger Publishing co, Inc. Malabar, Florida.)

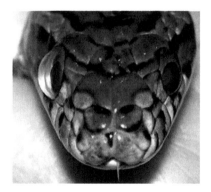

**Figure 10.28**  Mildly enlarged but still transparent spectacle in bullous spectaculopathy.

ance of the eye can be one of a protuberant opaque mass (Figure 10.27) or one where, while the spectacle is clearly distended, it remains transparent (Figure 10.28). The difficulty here is differentiating this from glaucoma, which would present in a similar manner in a non-spectacled animal, but with globe enlargement causing the clinical signs. Indeed in what is apparently the first mention of the condition in the literature, Drs Boniuk and Lusquette, used the term pseudobuphthalmos to indicate that it was not the globe that was enlarged but the spectacle alone [38]. They noted 'this apparent buphthalmos has often been misinterpreted as the result of an underlying glaucoma.' Martin Lawton has argued [39] that the term bullous spectaculopathy is inappropriate since the medical definition for bulla is an epithelial accumulation of fluid. The original Latin meaning, however, is a hollow thin-walled rounded prominence (consider for instance the tympanic bulla) and thus to my mind it would seem quite acceptable to use it for this distention of the spectacle, as Frye first did [40].

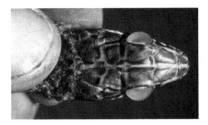

**Figure 10.29**   Snake with transient bullous spectaculopathy. (Reproduced with permission from Professor John E. Cooper.)

### Aetiopathogenesis

As we noted above the enclosure of the preocular tear film by the spectacle in snakes and some squamates, notably several geckos, means that nasolacrimal obstruction leads to swelling of the space between the cornea and the spectacle rather than epiphora. Later we will encounter instances where upwelling infection along the nasolacrimal duct results in abscessation between the cornea and spectacle, but here no infectious agent is involved and the problem is merely a mechanical swelling of the spectacle.

The nasolacrimal obstruction may be congenital with a developmental atresia of the duct, as has been reported in a blood python by Millichamp and colleagues [41]. More commonly it is caused by an acquired physical obstruction to the duct. In some cases [42], there is an infectious aetiology at its origin, in which case the condition should probably be termed a subspectacular abscess, as discussed further below.

Interestingly there are snakes which develop this condition just before ecdysis or shedding, when presumably the shed epithelium, which includes that of the nasolacrimal duct as well as the dermal epidermis, impedes tear drainage for a few days (Figure 10.29).

### Clinical management

Simple aspiration of the lacrimal fluid with a needle is possible but will only give temporary amelioration of the signs although this might be sufficient. The sample obtained is submitted for bacteriological culture and cytology. The fluid produced by the lacrimal and Harderian glands can be viscous precluding aspiration with a narrow-gauge needle as one might want to employ in such a situation. The standard treatment under general anaesthetic is to excise a ventral triangle of spectacle, allowing continual drainage of tears until the next shed (Figures 10.30 and 10.31). Such an approach requires microsurgery and should be performed by a specialist, ideally using an operating microscope, hence such cases are best referred to a veterinary ophthalmologist.

It is important to address the initial problem causing the nasolacrimal obstruction, normally an inflammatory aetiology associated with necrotic stomatitis. As noted above, Millichamp has reported a congenital nasolacrimal obstruction which required the formation of an artificial draining tract [43] but such cases are thankfully rare, since success in such surgery requires considerable surgical skill.

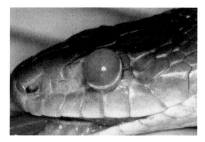

**Figure 10.30** Snake with bullous spectaculopathy anaesthetized for surgery. (Reproduced with permission from Dr Daniel Priehs.)

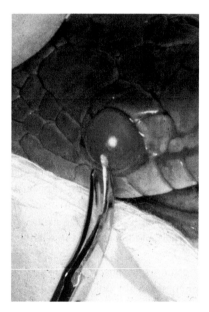

**Figure 10.31** Treatment by excision of a wedge ventrally. (Reproduced with permission from Dr Daniel Priehs.)

## Subspectacular abscessation

If obstruction of the nasolacrimal duct manifests in snakes as bullous spectaculopathy rather than the epiphora which would be seen in species without a spectacle, it is not surprising that infection of the nasolacrimal duct in snakes is seen as an abscess manifesting in the space between the cornea and spectacle, a subspectacular abscess.

### Clinical signs

Subspectacular abscesses can be easy to diagnose with a yellow mass in the ventral subspectacular space or in severe cases occupying the entire ocular surface (Figure 10.32), in which case differentiating it from a bullous spectaculopathy with opacity of

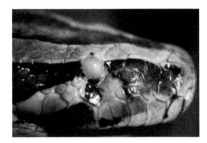

**Figure 10.32**   Snake with subspectacular abscessation.

the spectacle might be difficult. Conversely, some cases which initially appear as bullous spectaculopathy, are in fact infected, with inflammation and abscessation causing the nasolacrimal obstruction.

### Clinical management

As with bullous spectaculopathy, the optimal treatment is formation of a 30 degree ventral window in the spectacle though which the infected and inflammatory debris can be removed by irrigation. The purulent material can be caseous in nature and not fluid, as one might expect from say a cat bite abscess, rendering it significantly more difficult to remove from this narrow space than one might expect. As discussed earlier when considering periocular abscessation in reptiles, the involvement of heterophils in inflammatory processes in the lower vertebrates rather than neutrophils in mammals precludes the release of coagulative enzymes and thus results in what has been termed a fibriscess rather than an abscess [44].

Samples obtained from flushing the subspectacular space in such cases should be submitted for bacteriological culture and cytology, together with oral samples to assess the likelihood that necrotic stomatitis is the underlying cause of an ascending infection resulting in the ocular signs.

### Corneal ulceration

Corneal disease in reptiles may be a keratitis with or without attendant infection, traumatic ulceration or lipid deposition, and each of these diagnoses has different clinical signs.

### Clinical signs

Post-traumatic corneal ulcers in reptiles (other than snakes where the spectacle protects the cornea from such trauma) are an area where we can extrapolate from what is known in mammals more frequently seen in veterinary practice. Use of fluorecsein dye in exactly the same way as might be employed in an ulcerated canine or feline cornea, willl demarcate the extent of the ulcer and its depth (Figure 10.33).

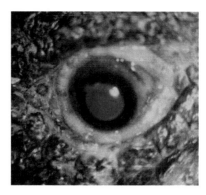

**Figure 10.33**   Post-traumatic corneal ulcer in a 38-year-old spur-thighed tortoise (*Testudo graeca*).

### Aetiopathogenesis

Most ulceration in reptiles is post-traumatic, although infection may be important in preventing healing or resulting in a more severe melting ulcer. In some older animals, and here it must be remembered that chelonia can have a very extended lifespan, geriatric lengthening of healing time may be an important factor precluding rapid healing.

### Clinical management

Staining a suspect corneal ulcer with a single drop of sodium fluorescein will allow appreciation of its extent. Other tests to complete the diagnostic work-up should include bacteriology and cytology, the latter obtained with a cytobrush smeared onto a clean slide, air-dried and stained with Diff-Quik as a modified Wright–Giemsa stain.

The three questions to ask of any ulcer are: (i) what is the cause of the ulcer? (ii) how deep is the ulcer? and (iii) is the ulcer healing? Most ulcers in reptiles have a history of a traumatic incident although some can be complicated by secondary infection. Many of these erosions are superficial but care must be taken given the thickness of the cornea in many reptiles kept in captivity. Corneal thickness in three leatherback turtles, for instance, ranged between 300 and 650 μm [45], the higher limit equating with the thickness of the canine cornea, but these are the largest eyes likely to be encountered among reptiles. Even a superficial ulcer in an iguana or a box turtle can involve a considerable proportion of the corneal thickness and so should be treated as an emergency.

Corneal ulcers usually heal rapidly, within 1 week, except where healing is delayed either because of an abnormality of the epithelial basement membrane as in recidivistic epithelial erosions in Boxer dogs [46] or in older animals as in Figure 10.33 where a traumatic ulcer has failed to heal in a 38-year-old tortoise. In such cases debridement of the redundant devitalized epithelium at the ulcer edge is important, probably followed by topical antibiotic to prevent secondary infection, although preservatives and stabilizers such as benzalkonium chloride have been shown to retard ulcer healing *in vitro* [47].

Third eyelid flaps can be used to protect eyes with ulcers but conjunctival pedicle flaps are difficult to fashion in small eyes such as those of the reptiles normally encountered in practice. Tear replacement drops, with a carbomer gel or sodium hyaluronate base, can be useful to ensure rapid healing.

### Corneal opacification

#### Clinical signs

While a long-standing corneal ulcer could cause corneal opacification, predominantly through pigmentation, lack of transparency is more normally related to a white discoloration of the cornea caused by either lipid, calcium or a proteinaceous deposit.

#### Aetiopathogenesis

Chelonia with a systemic circulating lipidaemia, either through an inherited dyslipoproteinaemia or a dietary hyperlipidaemia, have corneal lipidosis which is not dissimilar from that seen in the dog. The lesion appears a diffuse milky white colour (Figure 10.34) but at higher magnification individual lipid crystals may be evident.

A denser much more homogeneous white corneal lesion may be seen in reptiles, and particularly chelonia, after hibernation (Figure 10.35). Frye has reported that these can be dissolved using Kymar ointment, a preparation of alpha chymotrypsin, suggesting that this lesion is proteinaceous in nature [48].

#### Clinical management

In the same way that amelioration of lipid-related corneal pathology is difficult in companion mammals, these opacities, once formed, can be very taxing to resolve. The key feature in dealing with the lesions in reptiles as in other species is evaluating the underlying cause and removing it, with the hope that in time the corneal lipid deposition will gradually resolve. Assessing the individual's diet is essential.

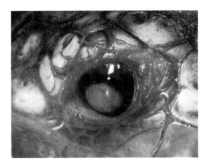

**Figure 10.34**   Red-footed tortoise with corneal lipidosis. (Reproduced with permission from Dr Stephen Barten.)

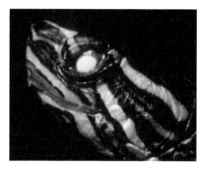

**Figure 10.35**   Terrapin with a post-hibernational corneal opacity. (Reproduced with permission from Dr Fredric Frye. Originally printed in *Biological and Surgical Aspects of Captive Reptile Husbandry, 2nd Ed.*, 1991, Krieger Publishing co, Inc. Malabar, Florida.)

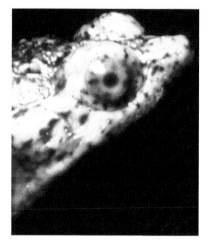

**Figure 10.36**   *Trionyx* turtle with uveitis manifesting as aqueous flare with irregular appearance of intraocular structures.

## Uveitis

### Clinical signs

Inflammation of the uveal tract, the iris anteriorly and the choroid posteriorly, together with the ciliary body, is rarely seen in reptiles. It can be a sign of systemic infection, as we saw to be the case with conjunctivitis. The main clinical signs of anterior uveitis are those of inflammatory cells in the anterior chamber of the eye with either flare in mild cases giving a hazy appearance to the iris (Figure 10.36), or more overt purulent deposits giving rise to hypopyon (Figure 10.37) [49,50]. It appears that pupil construction or miosis is less of a problem in reptiles than in mammals such as dogs and cats.

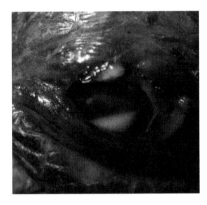

**Figure 10.37**   *Testudo graeca* tortoise with uveitis showing hypopyon.

### Aetiopathogenesis

The majority of cases in reptiles are associated with systemic Gram-negative infections, such as dissemination of *Pseudomas* sp. which led to uveitis with hypopyon in an Indonesian blue-tongued skink [51] or *Aeromonas* septicaemia as reported by Millichamp and Jacobson in the same review. *Klebsiella pneumoniae* infection was the cause of anterior uveitis, again manifest as hypopyon in a group of Tockay geckos [52]. Whether this association between septicaemia and intraocular inflammation shows the presence of infectious organisms in the eye is unclear. Circulating lipopolysaccharide, as would be seen in such a septicaemia, can lead to a breakdown of the blood–aqueous barrier with resultant flare without a frank intraocular infection, as least in rats when used as a laboratory model of uveitis, but the evidence base for this as the cause of reptile uveitic signs is shaky to say the least.

### Clinical management

Close examination with a slit lamp biomicroscope will show early signs of inflammatory cell circulation and fibrin deposition in uveitis. Because of the likelihood of association with systemic infection, blood culture should be undertaken as well as routine haematological and biochemical assessment. Parenteral antibiosis should ideally be based on bacteriological culture and sensitivity from a blood sample, but a broad-spectrum agent such as enrofloxacin or trimethoprim–sulphamethoxazole, considered 'old hat' by some but nevertheless effective, should be used before results of bacteriological investigations are available.

   As far as the eye is concerned topical steroids or non-steroidal agents are worthwhile even in the face of infection, since reducing the inflammatory processes in the eye is essential. Attempts at surgical removal of the purulent debris in a case of hyopyon has been reported in a case of fungal hypopyon but without long-term success; enucleation was eventually necessary [53].

In a mammal with anterior uveitis anti-inflammatory medication such as topical prednisone acetate would be supplemented with atropine as a parasympatholytic mydriatic to dilate the pupil. This is not effective in reptiles where, as we noted earlier, the iris muscle is striated. While topical non-depolarising muscle relaxant is sufficient to produce mydriasis in some lizards but not chelonia, it does not seem to be effective in situations where active inflammatory miosis is occurring. As noted earlier, aggressive miosis with synechia formation does not seem a pronounced sign in reptile uveitis, so this lack of effect is perhaps less concerning than we might otherwise consider it to be.

### Cataracts

#### Clinical signs

Mature blinding cataracts are readily visible as a white opacity through the pupil of the eye (Figure 10.38 and Figure 10.39). Immature cataracts may be more difficult to visualise without the use of ophthalmic equipment such as the direct ophthalmoscope and slit lamp biomicroscope, although if white they can be observed even at a distance (Figure 10.40). Incipient opacities in the lens are more difficult still to evaluate and the

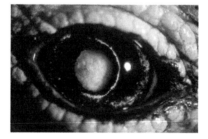

**Figure 10.38**   Blinding mature cataract in a tree monitor.

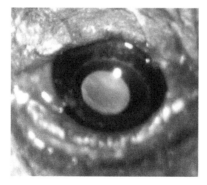

**Figure 10.39**   Mature cataract in tortoise eye.

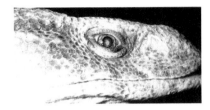

**Figure 10.40**    Immature developing cataract in a varanid monitor lizard.

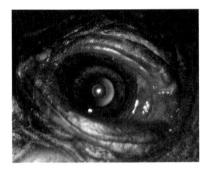

**Figure 10.41**    Nuclear sclerosis in a 40-year-old Aldabaran toroise.

most useful technique is retroillumination viewing against the red reflex using a direct ophthalmoscope at +10 D. Nuclear sclerosis, a normal change in the ageing eye, occurs where the central nucleus is compressed by the developing surrounding cortex, clearly visible as a ring in an otherwise clear lens (Figure 10.41).

### Aetiopathogenesis

As with any species there are several factors involved in the generation of lens opacity. As Taylor [54] suggested several years ago the 5 Ds of age-related cataract – daylight, diet, diabetes, drug and don't know – cover most of the bases! Now, with our understanding of genetic influences on cataract we can probably eliminate the 'don't know' and put DNA in its place since genetics seems to play a significant part in the aetiopathogenesis of age-related cataract as well as directly inherited cataract, which usually occurs at a younger age in a human or canine patient. This highlights two problems faced with many older captive reptiles developing cataract. Is this the result of an environmental or dietary factor or a genetic tendency to lens opacification? If the former, then we need to identify what changes should be made to the captive environment, and if the latter, then the animal should not be bred from, perpetuating a cataratogenic mutation.

The majority of published literature on cataracts in captive reptiles involves reports of surgery on individual animals [55,56]. Lawton has reported cataract as a possible sequel to freezing during hibernation [57]. Our research investigating cataracts in older *Testudo* species has shown that by the age of 35 most, if not all, tortoises of this genus have some degree of nuclear cataract without any reported hibernational catastrophes.

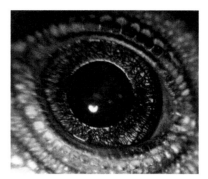

**Figure 10.42**   Immature posterior cortical cataract in *Physignathus leseuri.*

This is not surprising, since all animals appear to develop age-related lens opacities at around the same proportion of their life expectancy, as we have shown in companion mammals [58,59]. Lawton's cases, though, developed mature blinding cataracts which tended to clear over time, thus separating them from age-related lens opacities occurring later in life.

While we have no direct evidence for ultraviolet (UV) light causing cataracts in reptiles, the varanid monitor lizard in Figure 10.40 was housed very close to an ultraviolet light source. It is widely recognized in laboratory rodents, and by extrapolation to people, that UV light can lead to cataract formation through photo-oxidation of lens crystallin proteins. It is thus not surprising that UV may cause opacification in reptiles housed under quite powerful UV illumination in order to ensure that sufficient vitamin D3 is produced. The question might justifiably be asked, how much UV does each different species require? A useful website regarding this whole area is http://www.uvguide.co.uk.

We have examined the eyes of a number of bearded dragons (*Pogona vitticeps*) and Chinese water dragons (*Physignathus lesuerurii*) kept under the same UV irradiation at 350–450 $\mu$W/cm$^2$. The former is used, in its natural environment, to being exposed to considerable levels of UV irradiance while the latter, under a leaf canopy, is adapted for a substantially lower UV light level. Two different species from similar environments have been shown to have significantly different degrees of skin absorption of UV light [60] and we might expect the same from the different lenses of these two species. The forest dwelling lizard did have a significantly higher prevalence of nuclear and posterior cortical cataract (Figure 10.42) compared with the bearded dragon, a basking lizard. We presume the lens of the bearded dragon is adapted to high levels of UV.

Such a study is at best described as preliminary but still shows the importance of assessing the natural levels of UV experienced by each species and mirroring this as closely as possible in captivity.

## Clinical management

Cataract surgery by phacoemulsification has been performed successfully in several larger reptiles (Figure 10.43) [61,62].

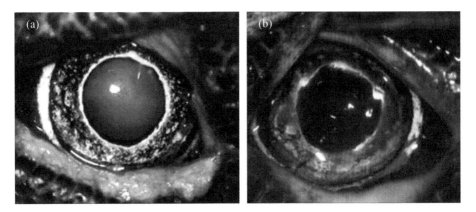

**Figure 10.43**   Savannah monitor eye (a) before and (b) after phacoemulsification surgery. (Reproduced with permission from Dr Carmen Colitz.)

## Glaucoma

While increased intraocular pressure has not been reported in reptiles, several papers have reported the normal intraocular pressure in breeds of tortoise and in alligators [63–66]. Significant differences in intraocular pressure occurred with sea turtles held in different positions [65] and in alligators of differing lengths [66]. All these reports determined intraocular pressure using the Tonopen applanation tonometer, too large for use in the smaller chelonia such as *Testudo graeca* or smaller lizards. Our initial studies with the Tonovet rebound tonometer suggest that it is a valuable tool in measuring intraocular pressure in these smaller reptiles.

Ramesh Tripathi's comprehensive account of aqueous outflow across the species allows us a valuable insight into the drainage pathways of each reptile group [67]. The differences between species of reptile occur because of variation in anterior chamber depth and the anatomy of the iridociliary cleft and ciliary musculature, this varying with the different mechanisms of accommodation, as discussed earlier.

Clearly the spectacle precludes the measurement of intraocular pressure in snakes by tonometry. It also means that assessment of globe size in these species can only be done using ultrasonography. Enlargement of the spectacle has to be the key differential diagnosis in snakes from an enlarged eye because of glaucoma, but since glaucoma in these species has yet to be reported it is difficult to give an assessment of techniques to differentiate buphthalmos and what has been called pseudobuphthalmos (see above). Another differential is megaglobus (see below) where the eye is abnormally large but visual and with a normal intraocular pressure.

## Microphthalmos and anophthalmos

### Clinical signs

As with any species, ocular congenital abnormalities may be encountered in reptiles and the most frequent are microphthalmos (Figure 10.44) and less commonly anophthalmos

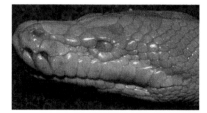

**Figure 10.44** Microphthalmos with opaque ocular surface in an albino kingsnake.

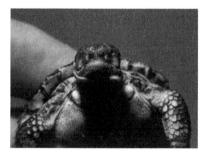

**Figure 10.45** Clinical anophthalmos in a tortoise incubated at too high a temperature.

(Figure 10.45). We term the latter clinical anophthalmos, as often a small remnant of pigmented tissue is visible at the orbital apex with magnification, and complete anophthalmos is rare. Visual dysfunction occurs in many cases ranging from total blindness in anophthalmic animals to mild visual impairment in microphthalmic animals. The key problem with blind animals is the difficulty in getting them to eat, since they are highly visually motivated feeders. A common problem also in moderate to severe cases is orbital infection, since the conjunctival sac is increased in size given the reduced globe diameter.

### Aetiopathogenesis

These congenital defects may be associated with egg incubation at too high a temperature; metabolism is inevitably increased and a relative hypoxia appears to occur resulting in abnormalities in globe development.

## Megaglobus

### Clinical signs

We have already noted that bullous spectaculopathy may appear as if the globe itself is enlarged, giving rise to the term pseudobuphthalmos. Globe enlargement can be seen in glaucoma when it would be accompanied by vision loss but has also been reported in eyes retaining vision in the Texas black rat snake in its leucistic form and then only in male individuals (Figure 10.46) [68].

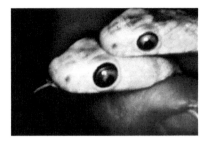

**Figure 10.46** Megaglobos in a male leucistic Texas black rat snake (below) compared with the female (above).

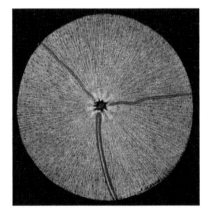

**Figure 10.47** Fundus of an Indian cobra from Wood's *Fundus Oculi of Birds* 1917.

## *Posterior segment lesions*

While the reptile retina has been the subject of a number of studies (the input of 'reptile' and 'retina' into the NCBI search engine pubmed yields 1089 hits!), reports of retinal disease are vanishingly rare in the literature. Casey Wood has a drawing of the fundus of an Indian cobra (Figure 10.47) drawn by the indefatigable and courageous Arthur Head while Johnson's monograph on the reptile eye, illustrated by the same gentleman, covers the reptile fundus in great detail [69]. The fascinating anatomical variation is in the retinal vasculature which varies markedly between species, demonstrating the widely varying evolutionary roots of different reptile classes.

Two exceptions to this paucity of data on retinal disease exist. The first is Lawton's report of post-hibernatinal freeze damage in *Testudo* retinas leading to blindness, although the relative contribution of retinal and central lesions to visual loss is difficult to assess with certainty [70]. The second is the retinal toxicity of mercury in alligators in the Florida everglades [71]. Changes in the electroretinogram were seen in mercury-intoxicated animals reflecting the high concentrations of the metal toxin in the retinas, optic nerves and optic tracts of affected individuals.

# References

1. Millichamp NJ, Jacobson ER, Wolf ED. Diseases of the eye and ocular adnexae in reptiles. J Am Vet Med Assoc 1983;183:1205–1212.
2. Lawton M. Reptilian ophthalmology. In: D Mader, ed. *Reptile Medicine and Surgery* 2nd edn. St Louis, Mo: Saunders, 2006.
3. Williams DL. Reptilian ophthalmology. In: D Mader, ed. *Reptile Medicine and Surgery* 1st edn. St Louis, Mo: Saunders, 1996.
4. Underwood G. The eye. In: C Gans, TS Parsons, eds. *Biology of the Reptilia* Vol 2B. London and New York: Academic Press, 1970; pp. 1–97.
5. Walls GL. *The Vertebrate Eye and its Adaptive Radiation.* Michigan: Cranbrook Institute of Science, 1942; pp. 607–641.
6. Duke Elder S. The eye in evolution. *System of Ophthalmology* Vol 1. London: Kimpton, 1958; pp. 353–395.
7. Citron MC, Pinto LH. Retinal image: larger and more luminous for a nocturnal than a diurnal lizards. Vision Res 1973;13:873–876.
8. Underwood op cit p. 89.
9. Minucci S, Chieffi Baccari G, di Matteo L. Histology, histochemistry, and ultrastructure of the harderian gland of the snake *Coluber viridiflavus.* J Morphol 1992;211:207–212.
10. Ott M. Visual accommodation in vertebrates: mechanisms, physiological response and stimuli. J Comp Physiol A Neuroethol Sens Neural Behav Physiol 2006;192:97–111.
11. Northmore DP, Granda AM. Ocular dimensions and schematic eyes of freshwater and sea turtles. Vis Neurosci 1991;7:627–635.
12. Abel JH, Ellis RA. Histochemical and electron microscopic observations on the salt secreting lachrymal glands of marine turtles. Am J Anat 1966;118:337–358.
13. Mead AW. Vascularity in the reptilian spectacle. Invest Ophthalmol 1976;15:587–591.
14. Roth LS, Kelber A. Nocturnal colour vision in geckos. Proc Biol Sci 2004;271(Suppl 6): S485–487.
15. Sillman AJ, Govardovskii VI, Röhlich P, Southard JA, Loew ER. The photoreceptors and visual pigments of the garter snake (*Thamnophis sirtalis*): a microspectrophotometric, scanning electron microscopic and immunocytochemical study. J Comp Physiol [A] 1997;181: 89–101.
16. Sillman AJ, Johnson JL, Loew ER. Retinal photoreceptors and visual pigments in Boa constrictor imperator. J Exp Zool 2001;290:359–365.
17. Malmström T, Kröger RH. Pupil shapes and lens optics in the eyes of terrestrial vertebrates. J Exp Biol 2006:209:18–25.
18. Grace MS, Woodward OM. Altered visual experience and acute visual deprivation affect predatory targeting by infrared-imaging Boid snakes. Brain Res 2001;919:250–258.
19. Murphy CJ, Howland HC. On the gekko pupil and Scheiner's disc. Vision Res 1986;26: 815–817.
20. Grace MS, Woodward OM. Altered visual experience and acute visual deprivation affect predatory targeting by infra-red-imaging Boid snakes. Brain Res 2001;1919: 250–258.
21. Grace MS, Woodward OM, Church DR, Catlisch G. Prey targeting by the infrared-imaging snake *Python*: effects of experimental and congenital visual deprivation. Behav Brain Res 2001;119:23–31.
22. Haverly JE, Kardong KV. Sensory deprivation effects on the predatory behaviour of the rattlesnake *Crotalus viridis oreganus.* Copeia 1996:419–428.
23. Kardong KV, Mackessey SP. The strike behaviour of a congenitally blind rattlesnake. J Herpetol 1991;25:208–211.

24. Frye FL. *Biomedical and surgical aspects of captive reptile husbandry.* Melbourne, FL: Kreiger Publishing, 1991; pp. 329–341.
25. Elkan E, Zwart P. The ocular disease of young terrapins caused by vitamin A deficiency. Pathol Vet 1967;4:201–222.
26. Jacobson ER, Popp JA, Shields RP, Gaskin JM. Poxlike skin lesions in captive caimans. J Am Vet Med Assoc 1979;175:937–940.
27. Lackovich JK, Brown DR, Homer BL, Garber RL, Mader DR, Moretti RH, Patterson AD, Herbst LH, Oros J, Jacobson ER, Curry SS, Klein PA. Association of herpesvirus with fibro-papillomatosis of the green turtle *Chelonia mydas* and the loggerhead turtle *Caretta caretta* in Florida. Dis Aquat Organ 1999;37:89–97.
28. Jacobson ER, Gaskin JM, Roelke M, Greiner EC, Allen J. Conjunctivitis, tracheitis, and pneumonia associated with herpesvirus infection in green sea turtles. J Am Vet Med Assoc 1986;189:1020–1023.
29. Cooper JE, McClelland MH, Needham JR. An eye infection in laboratory lizards associated with an *Aeromonas* species. Lab Anim 1980;14:149.
30. Huchzermeyer FW, Langlet E, Putterill JP. An outbreak of chlamydiosis in farmed Indopacvific crocodiles (*Crocodylus porosus*). J S Afr Vet Assoc 2008;79:99–100.
31. Tangredi BP, Evans RH. Organochlorine pesticides associated with ocular, nasal, or otic infection in the eastern box turtle (*Terrapene carolina carolina*). J Zoo Wildl Med 1997;28:97–100.
32. Abou-Madi N, Kern TJ. Squamous cell carcinoma associated with a periorbital mass in a veiled chameleon (*Chamaeleo calyptratus*). Vet Ophthalmol 2002;5:217–220.
33. Schumacher J, Pellicane CP, Heard DJ, Voges A. Periorbital abscess in a chameleon (*Chameleon jacksonii*). Vet Comp Ophthalmol 1996;6:30–33.
34. Allgoewer I, Göbel T, Stockhaus C, Schaeffer EH. Dacryops in a red-eared slider (*Chrysemys scripta elegans*): case report. Vet Ophthalmol 2002;5:231–234.
35. Whittaker CJG, Schumacher J, Bennett AR *et al.* Orbital varix in a green iguana (*Iguana iguana*). Vet Comp Ophthalmol 1997;7:101–104.
36. Montali RJ. Comparative pathology of inflammation in the higher vertebrates (reptiles, birds and mammals). J Comp Pathol 1988;99:1–26.
37. Hardon T, Fledelius B, Heegaard S. Keratoacanthoma of the spectacle in a Boa constrictor. Vet Ophthalmol 2007;10:320–322.
38. Boniuk M, Lusquette GF. Leucocoria and pseudobuphthalmos in snakes. Invest Ophthalmol 1963;2:283.
39. Lawton M. Reptilian ophthalmology. In: D Mader, ed. *Reptile Medicine and Surgery* 2nd edn. St Louis, Mo: Saunders, 2006; p. 340.
40. Frye FL. *Biomedical and surgical aspects of captive reptile husbandry.* Melbourne, FL: Kreiger Publishing, 1991; pp. 329–341.
41. Millichamp NJ, Jacobson ER, Dziezyc J. Conjunctivoralostomy for treatment of an occluded lacrimal duct in a blood python. J Am Vet Med Assoc 1986;189:1136–1138.
42. Cullen CL, Wheler C, Grahn BH. Diagnostic ophthalmology. Bullous spectaculopathy in a king snake. Can Vet J 2000;41:327–328.
43. Millichamp NJ, Jacobson ER, Wolf ED. Diseases of the eye and ocular adnexae in reptiles. J Am Vet Med Assoc 1983;183:1205–1212.
44. Huchzermeyer FW, Cooper JE. Fibriscess, not abscess, resulting from a localised inflammatory response to infection in reptiles and birds. Vet Rec 2000;147:515–517.
45. Brudenall DK, Schwab IR, Fritsches KA Ocular morphology of the Leatherback sea turtle (*Dermochelys coriacea*). Vet Ophthalmol 2008;11:99–110.
46. Murphy CJ, Marfurt CF, McDermott A, Bentley E, Abrams GA, Reid TW, Campbell S. Spontaneous chronic corneal epithelial defects (SCCED) in dogs: clinical features, innerva-

tion, and effect of topical SP, with or without IGF-1. Invest Ophthalmol Vis Sci 2001;42: 2252–2261.

47. Ayaki M, Yaguchi S, Iwasawa A, Koide R. Cytotoxicity of ophthalmic solutions with and without preservatives to human corneal endothelial cells, epithelial cells and conjunctival epithelial cells. Clin Experiment Ophthalmol 2008;36:553–559.

48. Frye FL. *Biomedical and surgical aspects of captive reptile husbandry*. Melbourne, FL: Kreiger Publishing, 1991; pp. 329–341.

49. Bonney CH, Hartfiel DA, Schmidt RE. *Klebsiella pseumoniae* infection with secondary hypopyon in Tokay gecko lizards. J Am Vet Med Assoc 1978;173:1115–1116.

50. Tomson FN, McDonnell SE, Wolf ED. Hypopyon in a tortoise. J Am Vet Med Assoc 1976;169:942.

51. Millichamp NJ, Jacobson ER, Wolf ED. Diseases of the eye and ocular adnexae in reptiles. J Am Vet Med Assoc 1983;183:1205–1212.

52. Bonney CH, Hartfiel DA, Schmidt RE. *Klebsiella pneumoniae* infection with secondary hypopyon in tokay gecko lizards. J Am Vet Med Assoc 1978;173:1115–1116.

53. Zwart P, Verwer MAJ, DeVried GA *et al.* Fungal infection of the eyes of the snake *Epicrates chendra maurus*: enucleation under halothane narcosis. J Small An Pract 1973;14:773.

54. Robman L, Taylor H. External factors in the development of cataract. Eye 2005;19: 1074–1082.

55. Colitz CM, Lewbart G, Davidson MG. Phacoemulsification in an adult Savannah monitor lizard. Vet Ophthalmol 2002;5:207–209.

56. Kelly TR, Walton W, Nadelstein B, Lewbart GA. Phacoemulsification of bilateral cataracts in a loggerhead sea turtle (*Caretta caretta*). Vet Rec 2005;156:774–777.

57. Lawton MPC, Stokes LC. Post-hibernational blindness in tortoises (*Testudo* spp.) In: ER Jacobson, ed. Third International Colloquium on Pathology of Reptiles and Amphibians. Orlando FL 1989.

58. Williams DL, Heath MF. Prevalence of feline cataract: results of a cross-sectional study of 2000 normal animals, 50 cats with diabetes and one hundred cats following dehydrational crises. Vet Ophthalmol 2006;9:341–349.

59. Williams DL, Heath MF, Wallis C. Prevalence of canine cataract: preliminary results of a cross-sectional study. Vet Ophthalmol 2004;7:29–35.

60. Carman EN, Ferguson GW, Gehrmann WH, Chen TC, Holick MF. Photobiosynthetic opportunity and ability for UVB generated vitamin D synthesis in free-living house geckos (*Hemidactylus turcicus*) and Texas spiny lizards (*Sceloporus olivaceous*). Copeia 2000: 245–250. Available online at http://www.reptileuvinfo.com/docs/vitamin-d-house-geckos-texas-spiny.pdf

61. Colitz CM, Lewbart G, Davidson MG. Phacoemulsification in an adult Savannah monitor lizard. Vet Ophthalmol 2002;5:207–209.

62. Kelly TR, Walton W, Nadelstein B, Lewbart GA. Phacoemulsification of bilateral cataracts in a loggerhead sea turtle (*Caretta caretta*). Vet Rec 2005;156:774–777.

63. Selmi AL, Mendes GM, MacManus C. Tonometry in adult yellow-footed tortoises (*Geochelone denticulata*). Vet Ophthalmol 2003;6:305–307.

64. Selmi AL, Mendes GM, McManus C, Arrais P. Intraocular pressure determination in clinically normal red-footed tortoise (*Geochelone carbonaria*). J Zoo Wildl Med 2002; 33:58–61.

65. Chittick B, Harms C. Intraocular pressure of juvenile loggerhead sea turtles (*Caretta caretta*) held in different positions. Vet Rec 2001;149:587–589.

66. Whittaker CJ, Heaton-Jones TG, Kubilis PS, Smith PJ, Brooks DE, Kosarek C, Mackay EO, Gelatt KN. Intraocular pressure variation associated with body length in young American alligators (*Alligator mississippiensis*). Am J Vet Res 1995;56:1380–1383.

67. Tripathi RG. Comparative physiology and anatomy of the aqueous outflow pathway. In: Davson H, Graham LT Jr, eds. *The Eye*, Vol 5. New York and London: Academic Press, 1974.

68. Bechtel HB, Bechtel E. Genetics of color mutations in the snake *Elaphe obselata*. J Hered 1985;76:7.

69. Johnston GL. Contributions to the comparative anatomy of the reptilian and the amphibian eye, chiefly based on ophthalmological examination. Philos Trans R Soc Lond B Biol Sci 1927;215:315–353 available online at http://www.jstor.org/stable/92111.

70. Lawton MPC, Stoakes LC. Post-hibernation blindness in tortoises (*Testudo* sp.) In: Jacobson ER, ed. Third International Colloquium on Pathology of Reptiles and Amphibians. Orlando Fl 1989.

71. Heaton-Jones TG, Homer BL, Heaton-Jones DL, Sundlof SF. Mercury distribution in American alligators (*Alligator mississippiensis*) in Florida. J Zoo Wildl Med 1997;28:62–70.

# Chapter 11

# The amphibian eye

Perhaps more than any other group of animals covered in this volume, amphibians have been the subject of research in vision. From a basic science question such as the organisation of ocular reflexes and their neurological sequelae [1] to behavioural issues, such as the role of amphibian vision in mate choice [2], researchers have investigated the amphibian visual system in great depth. Yet when it comes to assessing the amphibian eye in disease, relatively little research has been undertaken on captive animals and virtually none on wild populations. Given the parlous state of amphibian conservation worldwide [3,4], this is certainly a worrying lacuna. Ocular pathology in wild-caught amphibians does give rise for concern with congenital defects such as anophthalmos seen [5]. While the number of cases is small, one would not expect to see any blind animals in the wild, since their survival would be severely compromised. Eye disease in captive amphibians is important for their welfare and also for the health status of animals reintroduced into the wild, the prime aim, it would be hoped, of any and all captive breeding programmes [6].

## Anatomy and physiology of the amphibian eye

The very fact of being amphibian, living in both aquatic and terrestrial environments (hence the term amphi bios – double life), means that the amphibian eye has to be adapted to both visual niches. How does the eye of the developing tadpole cope with a sudden move from an aquatic niche to a terrestrial one where its eye, emetropic underwater, becomes exceptionally myopic in air [7]? In that way the amphibian visual system seems very far from our own. And yet the amphibian eye has been widely used as an experimental model of vision in higher animals.

In the same way that amphibians have evolved from fish and adapted to a more terrestrial existence in most species, the eye has adapted also. Eyelids protect the ocular surface to some extent and the Harderian gland provides tears to moisten the corneal surface. The globe is almost spherical with the cornea and sclera having the same radius of curvature. Tadpoles of the anura and urodela orders have a purely fibrous sclera; after metamorphosis many develop a cup of hyaline cartilage providing stablisation for the

*Ophthalmology of Exotic Pets*, First Edition. David L. Williams.
© 2012 David Williams. Published 2012 by Blackwell Publishing Ltd.

enlarging eye and an insertion for the rectus muscles. The most important of these is the retractor oculi, essential in pulling the eye in and down to form an integral part of the roof of the buccal cavity during swallowing. The cornea of many larval amphibian stages is duplex, as seen in the fish, with a dermal 'spectacle' and a deeper dural cornea, while in the adult it has the form seen in higher vertebrates. The anterior chamber of the adult is deep with the spherical lens situated almost centrally in the globe but moving forward by the action of the protractor lentis muscle, which is central in accommodation in these eyes (Figure 11.1). The iris is thin and well vascularised as shown in the beautiful work of Dame Ida Mann with the constricted pupil taking a multitude of differing shapes across the various species: a horizontal slit in *Hyla* species, a vertical one in *Hylates* and a heart-shaped one in *Bominator* (Figure 11.2). While there is striated iridal muscle as in

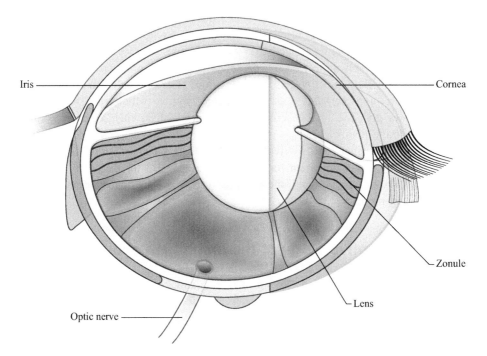

**Figure 11.1**  The amphibian eye.

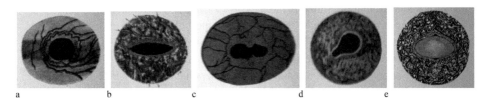

**Figure 11.2**  Different amphibian iris patterns and pupil shapes. (a) *Triturus torosus* (Californian newt). (b) *Bufo marinus* (Marine toad). (c) *Hyperlius horstockii* (Horstock's tree frog). (d) *Caloptochephalus quoyi* (Gay's frog). (e) *Hyla coerula* (White's tree frog). From Ida Mann's beautiful monograph, Iris patterns in the vertebrates. Transactions of the Zoological Society of London 1931;XXI(IV):355–412.

all lower vertebrates, considerable autonomous activity allows the pupil to constrict directly upon light stimulation, with contraction even said to occur in the enucleated eye [8]! Given such information, the diagnostic power of the amphibian pupillary light reflex with regard to visual function must be regarded with some considerable caution.

## What do amphibians see?

The importance of vision to amphibian genera is as varied as the animals themselves. The primitive caecilians and the retrograde subterranean and blind cave salamanders such as *Proteus anguilis* have degenerate eyes which can still sense light and dark but have no perception of form or movement. Intriguingly *P. anguilis* has light-sensitive skin with the photopigment melanopsin present in dermal melanophores [9].

Most anurans and salamanders, however, employ vision as their primary sense in prey location, primarily using a sit-and-wait strategy. The tree frog *Hyla cinerea*, for instance, has been shown to obtain 88% of its prey after visual detection and a short pursuit [10]. It used to be thought that amphibians could not detect stationary prey items but only moving objects. Put a frog in a room with dead insects on pins, so it is said, and the animal will die of starvation [11]. While movement of prey is an important stimulus to prey-catching behaviour, numerous amphibians use other cues as well as movement in prey detection and identification. A complex interaction of velocity, size and orientation is important in determining amphibian reaction to passing prey items. Even more intriguing, research has shown that *Bufo* toads reject bumblebees as noxious rather than prey items, by sight alone [12]. Tadpole schooling is to some degree vision-dependent although the lateral line system also plays an important part in orientation: individuals of some species such as *Xenopus laevis* orientate themselves in a parallel manner in the school more exactly in light, but in the dark, tight schooling still occurs. Others, such as *Phrynomerus annectens*, school during the day but disperse in the dark [13].

When we come to examine depth perception, so important in prey capture for many species, different amphibians vary considerably. Those with small eyes placed laterally have little in the way of binocular vision, while those with large protruberant eyes, such as many anurans and several salamanders, have almost 360-degree visual fields with significant overlap of the right and left eye vision. Indeed binocular vision or stereopsis has been shown to be important for prey capture in *Rana* and *Bufo* [14]. Such information is important if considering unilateral enucleation after trauma or neoplasia – anurans with one eye ablated are significantly compromised at making accurate movements towards prey and avoiding barriers [15].

The other mechanism for depth perception is accommodation. In amphibians this occurs through change in position of the lens, with a forward movement effected by two protractor muscles in anurans while salamanders have only one and here the effect of accommodation is less than 5 dioptres. Indeed experiments where lens accommodation is minimised show little change in behaviour and prey capture success, suggesting that accommodation plays little part in depth perception in these species.

The bright colours employed as breeding signals by amphibians such as male newts would suggest that colour vision exists in these species. It is often wavelengths which

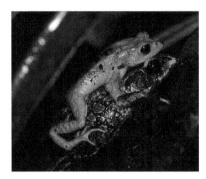

**Figure 11.3**   Striking colour differences between genders in amphibians such as the golden toad (*Bufo periglenes*) show the importance of colour vision in some of these species.

we cannot ourselves detect that may be the most important in other species, and vision in the ultraviolet range is present and may be important in many amphibians [16]. Colour vision is difficult to assess in amphibians, but behavioural work on *Xenopus* and *Rana* tadpoles shows two different responses. One is phototactic with a bimodal spectral sensitivity with maxima at 560 µm and at 460 µm (green and blue wavelengths respectively) while an optomotor response to the stimulus of a rotating set of grid lines has one stimulus maximum at 650 µm, well into the red hues of the visible light spectrum. Adult amphibians may have significantly different visual responses to light of different wavelengths from those of their larval progenitors and different species, with varying visual ecologies (some existing in deeper water where spectral maxima of ambient light are different from those of terrestrial species for instance), have quite different visual capabilities.

Indeed some amphibians manifest no sexual dimorphism with regard to their colour and in these generally nocturnally breeding animals there is no evidence for overt colour vision. In diurnally breeding species such as *Bufo canorus* (the Yosemite toad) and *Bufo periglenes* (the golden toad), striking sexual colour differences are evident, this being indirect evidence for colour vision in these animals (Figure 11.3).

# Diseases of the amphibian eye

## Corneal ulceration

### Clinical signs

The protuberant nature of many anuran eyes and the limited protection provided by the amphibian eyelids renders the amphibian eye more liable to corneal ulceration than that of many other animal groups. The limited thickness of the amphibian cornea also means that any corneal erosion or ulceration can potentially be dangerous for the integrity of the eye. The use of fluorescein dye can, as with any species, determine the extent of ulceration with regard to its lateral spread and its depth (Figure 11.4).

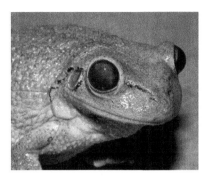

**Figure 11.4**   Corneal ulceration demonstrated by fluorescein dye uptake.

## Aetiopathogenesis

Corneal ulcers in amphibians, as in any species, are commonly traumatic in origin as noted above, but infection may also be a predisposing or a complicating factor, which it is important to take into account. Corneal oedema can occur as a result of loss of epithelial integrity but can in some instances be a contributory cause of ulceration with a bleb of water causing a bulla of epithelium which can then rupture, giving an ulcer which fails to heal precisely because of the oedematous underlying stroma.

## Clinical management

The use of topical antibiotics must be treated with caution in amphibians since systemic absorption across their highly permeable skin can result in systemic toxicity. Thus eye drops such as fluoroquinolones or chloramphenicol are to be preferred, for instance, over aminoglycosides which could result in renal toxicity. Third eyelid flaps can be used in certain species, but in many the third eyelid reflex is strong enough to tear out sutures in the delicate epithelial margin of the nictitating membrane. Where underlying stromal oedema is precluding rapid corneal healing it can be very difficult to resolve matters. In the thicker canine cornea a thermal keratoplasty may be in order, but in the thin cornea of most amphibians such a treatment is likely to lead to corneal perforation, and is thus to be avoided.

## UV-mediated ocular pathology

### Clinical signs

Ultraviolet irradiation-mediated ocular surface damage may be seen either as an inflammatory keratitis or more frequently a degenerative white opacity which can be distinguished from lipid keratopathy in that is is a sparser more crystalline opacity (Figure 11.5 – compare with Figure 11.7). Intraocular changes on UV irradiation are most commonly characterised by opacification of the lens. Tadpoles maintained in high levels of UV-B showed skin ulceration and a significantly higher level of cataract formation than

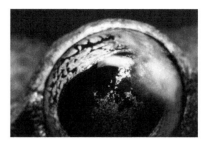

**Figure 11.5**   UV keratopathy.

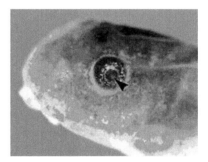

**Figure 11.6**   Cataract formation in tadpole kept in high UV-B radiation.

those kept at ambient UV levels (Figure 11.6) [17]. Whether cataracts occurring in amphibians in the wild can be attributed to increased levels of UV irradiation, especially in these times of atmospheric ozone depletion is difficult to say, but given that many occur in amphibians experimentally exposed to UV-B radiation, it might be reasonable to ascribe such changes to UV irradiation. The same could be said for idiopathic cataract in amphibians kept in captivity under UV light to optimise their vitamin D production. Amphibians in the wild have been shown to be affected by UV [18] but research has generally been focused on developmental abnormalities in tadpole larvae and not on defects in adults exposed to high levels of ultraviolet irradiation.

## Lipid keratopathy

### Clinical signs

Perhaps the most common ocular condition seen in captive amphibians is that of lipid keratopathy (Figures 11.7–11.9). Presenting as a white opacity in the cornea, more often than not protruding from the corneal surface, lipid deposition in the cornea is not difficult to diagnose. Most reports in the literature concern Cuban tree frogs (*Osteopilus septen-trionalis*) or White's free frog (*Litoria versicolor*) which have been kept in captivity for a considerable period although any amphibian can potentially be so affected [19]. Differential diagnoses might include corneal scarring or inflammatory cell infiltration but the raised surface and intense white colouration of the lesion is pathognomic.

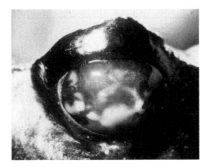

**Figure 11.7**   Lipid keratopathy in an American bullfrog.

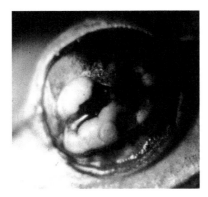

**Figure 11.8**   Lipid keratopathy in a White's tree frog.

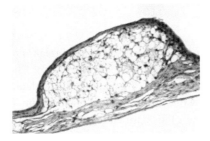

**Figure 11.9**   Histological section of cornea with lipid keratopathy. (Reproduced courtesy of Professor Peer Zwart.)

## Aetiopathogenesis

Initially this was considered to occur only in female frogs with the conjecture being that animals ready to spawn but unable to find an appropriate place in a captive environment, had an elevated blood lipid level for an unusually long time. In such cases lipid is deposited in the cornea secondary to this circulating lipid abnormality.

In fact lipid deposits occur in many body tissues and the condition is seen in male as well as female amphibians, so the hypothesis that the lipid deposition relates to unsuccessful spawning cannot be true in all cases, although it may be an important factor in some, or indeed many, cases.

Lipid levels in affected amphibians and normal control animals have been reported with affected individuals having serum cholesterol of $17.4 \pm 16.1$ mmol/l while unaffected animals had levels of $5.3 \pm 6.8$ mmol/l [20]. An experimental study reported in the same review fed Cuban tree frogs fed crickets containing 0.1% cholesterol on a dry matter basis. Corneal lipid arcus developed in eight animals fed the high cholesterol diet, four females and four males, while three females on a regular diet also developed lipid lesions in their corneas. The animals with corneal arcus had significantly higher circulating cholesterol levels than unaffected animals ($27.3 \pm 19.8$ mmol/l vs. $16.5 \pm 20.4$ mmol/l respectively but the ratio of VLDL and LDL to HDL and levels of VLDL, HDL and triclyceride did not differ between affected and unaffected animals.

The relevance of this dietary study is that large captive anurans may be fed newborn mice which, if they have already suckled, as most have, will have a high lipid content through ingested milk. Having said that frogs fed on more natural diets have been noted with the condition also.

### Clinical management

Attempts to reduce circulating lipid levels are generally somewhat fruitless although allowing females to find an acceptable place to spawn may be very important in relevant cases. Superficial keratectomy can be performed to remove the lipid but the thin nature of most amphibian corneas renders such surgery best performed under an operating microscope by a specialised ophthalmic surgeon.

### Periocular dermal ulceration

### Clinical signs

Fungal dermal conditions are well recognised in amphibians and these can cause particularly severe disease in the periocular area (Figure 11.10). Chromomycosis and phycomycosis lead to skin ulceration with or without skin reddening through inflammation, while *Saprolegnia* gives a white fluffy deposit on the skin. These are skin conditions rather than strictly ocular ones, thus dermatological texts should be consulted in dealing with them.

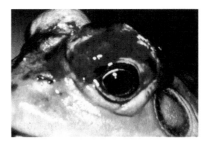

**Figure 11.10**   Chromomycosis involving the upper eyelid in a bullfrog.

### Aetiopathogenesis

A number of fungal organisms can be involved including the ascomycetes *Fonsecaea*, *Philalophora* and *Cladosporium*, while phycomycosis is caused by the phycomycetes *Absidia*, *Mucor* or *Rhizopus*. Defining the exact agent is not important since the treatment (see below) is similar. Note that these are not related to the chytrid fungus *Batrachochytrium dendrobatidis* which is causing dramatic declines in amphibian populations in the wild globally.

### Clinical management

Treatment for these dermal fungi is normally immersion in solutions of malchite green for periods of up to 5 minutes, although where the lesion is periocular treatment by laying gauze swabs soaked in medication over the area but not touching the ocular surface is to be preferred.

## Cataracts

Opacities in the lens may be noted as incidental findings, particularly in older animals (Figure 11.11) or, as noted above, possibly secondary to ultraviolet irradiation (Figure 11.6). Cataracts have been reported as occurring after 5% dextrose administration as supportive therapy in dendrobatid frogs but these opacities were reversible. Cataracts are currently reported to be a serious disease in farmed tiger frogs, *Rana tigerina rugulosa*, in China [21], although their aetiology is as yet unclear.

## Uveitis

### Clinical signs

The classic signs of intraocular inflammation are miosis, breakdown of the blood–aqueous barrier with fibrin, inflammatory cells or frank haemorrhage in the anterior chamber, hyperaemia of both intraocular and episcleral vasculature, and pain. We cannot

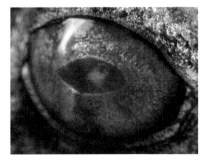

**Figure 11.11**   Incidental finding of lens opacity.

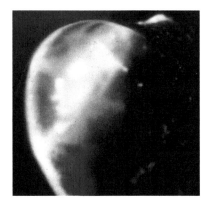

**Figure 11.12**   Uveitis associated with Gram-negative septicaemia.

tell in amphibians the degree to which this last feature is experienced, but the cases in which uveitis has been reported in amphibians demonstrate the other classic signs of uveitis [22–24].

### Aetiopathogenesis

Any traumatic episode can give rise to uveitis through damage to intraocular tissues and the amphibian is no exception here. In many other species from cats to horses, systemic infections can give rise to uveitis. In the mammals we deal with regularly most of these uveitiogens are viruses, such as feline infectious peritonitis or canine adenovirus, or parasites such as *Ehrlichia* or *Leishmania*. The amphibian seems particularly prone to its iris acting as a target tissue for the effects of Gram-negative septicaemia. Thus any amphibian with the classic signs of uveitis should be evaluated for bacterial septicaemia. Uveitis associated with Gram-negative septicaemia has been reported by Brooks and co-workers in fire-bellied toads (Figure 11.12) [22] and Olson and colleagues in leopard frogs [23], but the underlying mechanism has yet to be fully elucidated. Is it the same one that causes uveitis in mice injected with endotoxin? There the lipopolysaccharide breaks down the blood–aqueous barrier and precipitates an intraocular inflammatory response [25]. Or is it related to direct bacterial attack on iris tissues? We know that in septicaemic anurans the skin is a sentinel organ, with hyperaemia giving 'red leg'. It appears that the iris, with its substantial vascular network, is a second sentinel tissue, reacting to systemic Gram-negative infection. In the third case of uveitis reported, this time in Asian horned frogs with a rhabditid nematode infection, the keratitis, uveitis and encephalitis noted were associated with intralesional parasites [24]. Again it is difficult to know if the inflammation is an immune reaction specifically against the parasite or a more innate immune response to irritation experienced as the larvae migrate through the tissues. Whatever the situation, these cases show the importance of a full clinical examination when presented with an amphibian with ocular inflammation.

### Clinical management

Given the systemic disease in most of these uveitic animals, the key task is isolation of these animals from any in-contact animals and careful examination of those apparently healthy individuals. Blood culture from affected animals and post-mortem of any deceased cases is essential. Treatment of affected animals, and probably also in-contact stock with parenteral antibiotic, such as enrofloxacin (5–10 mg/kg) subcutaneously or intramuscularly once daily, or oxytetracycline injected by the same route at 25 mg/kg, is probably the best option. Small stock may best be medicated with a bath of an antibiotic, such as rifampicin at 25 mg/l, or treatments conventional to amphibian keepers but less so to veterinarians such as baths of methylene blue at 3 mg/l or malachite green at 150 μg/l.

## Glaucoma

### Clinical signs

As with any species, a rise in intraocular pressure in an amphibian may manifest itself with blindness, corneal oedema and, in severe cases, globe enlargement. Episcleral vessel congestion appears not to be a consistent finding in amphibians with glaucoma, maybe because the vasculature is too narrow in calibre to be readily visible. The small size of the amphibian eye and the consequent thinness of the sclera, render globe enlargement or buphthalmos a sign occurring rapidly in glaucoma in these individuals (Figure 11.13).

### Aetiopathogenesis

Amphibian glaucoma has not been investigated in detail, as it occurs rarely in these species. It would appear that most cases occur secondary to intraocular inflammation, where inflammatory debris occludes the drainage angle.

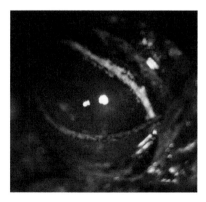

**Figure 11.13** Glaucoma with buphthalmos in a toad.

### Clinical management

We have no evidence for the medical management of raised intraocular pressure in amphibians. Given the importance of carbonic anhydrase in acid–base balance and muscle contraction in amphibians [26] and the rapid absorption of such drugs across the amphibian skin, the use of topical or systemic carbonic anhydrase inhibitors is not to be recommended.

## Enucleation

While one might think that the optimal surgical treatment for a painful blind amphibian eye is enucleation, as in a companion mammal species, amphibians have no hard palate, and as such the ventral surface of the globe forms part of the dorsal buccal cavity. This means that a frog or toad retropulses its eye very slightly into its buccal cavity to provide sufficient intraoral pressure to facilitate swallowing. An amphibian which has been enucleated, therefore, has great difficulty in swallowing, and as such enucleation is not to be recommended in these species. Evisceration and the implantation of an intraocular prosthesis might be preferable, although to this author's knowledge this technique has not been reported in the literature.

## Conclusion

The differences between the diagnosis, aetiology and treatment of conditions such as uveitis and glaucoma in amphibians show just how different these exotic species can be compared with the cats, dogs and horses we deal with on a daily basis. It is to be regretted that in these species where we need more species-specific information, so little exists currently in the veterinary literature. And yet there are substantial similarities too, so with care the knowledge we have of the mammalian eye can be extrapolated to the frog, toad or newt: the challenge is working out where extrapolation is appropriate and where it is not!

## References

1. Straka H, Dieringer N. Basic organization principles of the VOR: lessons from frogs. Prog Neurobiol 2004;73:259–309.
2. Cummings ME, Bernal XE, Reynaga R, Rand AS, Ryan MJ. Visual sensitivity to a conspicuous male cue varies by reproductive state in *Physalaemus pustulosus* females. J Exp Biol 2008; 211:1203–1210.
3. Rohr JR, Raffel TR, Romansic JM, McCallum H, Hudson PJ. Evaluating the links between climate, disease spread, and amphibian declines. Proc Natl Acad Sci U S A 2008;105: 17436–17441.
4. Pennisi E. Amphibian decline. Life and death play out on the skins of frogs. Science 2009;326: 507–508.

5. Schoff PK, Johnson CM, Schotthoefer AM, Murphy JE, Lieske C, Cole RA, Johnson LB, Beasley VR. Prevalence of skeletal and eye malformations in frogs from north-central United States: estimations based on collections from randomly selected sites. J Wildl Dis 2003;39: 510–521.

6. Griffiths RA, Pavajeau L. Captive breeding, reintroduction, and the conservation of amphibians. Conserv Biol 2008;22:852–861.

7. Hoskins SG. Metamorphosis of the amphibian eye. J Neurobiol 1990;21:970–989.

8. Brown-Sequard CE. Recherches de experimentales sur l'influence excitatrice de la lumiere, du froid et du la chaleur sur l'iris, dans les cinq classes d'animaux vertebres. J Physiol Homme Anim 1859;2:281–294.451–460.

9. Kos M, Bulog B, Szél A, Röhlich P. Immunocytochemical demonstration of visualpigments in the degenerate retinal and pineal photoreceptors of the blind cavesalamander (*Proteus anguinus*). Cell Tissue Res 2001;303:15–25.

10. Freed AN. Prey selection and feeding behavior of the green treefrog (*Hyla Cinerea*). Ecology 1980;61:461–465.

11. Ingle DJ. Prey-catching behavior of anurans toward moving and stationary objects. Vision Res 1971;S3:447–456.

12. Brower LP, Brower JVZ, Westcott PW. Experimental studies of mimicry. 5. The reactions of toads (*Bufo terrestris*) to bumblebees (*Bombus americanorum*) and their robberfly mimics (*Mallophora bomboides*), with a discussion of aggressive mimicry. Am Nat 1960;878: 343–355.

13. Channing A. Life histories of frogs in the Namib desert. Zoologica Africana 1976;11: 299–312.

14. Ingle D. Spatial vision in anurans. In: KV Fite, ed. *The Amphibian Visual System*. New York: Academic Press, 1976; pp. 119–140.

15. Collett T. Steropsis in toads. Nature 1977;267:349–351.

16. Shi Y, Yokoyama S. Molecular analysis of the evolutionary significance of ultraviolet vision in vertebrates. Proc Natl Acad Sci U S A 2003;100:8308–8313.

17. Novales Flamarique I, Ovaska K, Davis TM. UV-B induced damage to the skin and ocular system of amphibians. Biol Bull 2000;199:187–188.

18. Bancroft BA, Baker NJ, Blaustein AR. A meta-analysis of the effects of ultraviolet B radiation and its synergistic interactions with pH, contaminants, and disease on amphibian survival. Conserv Biol 2008;22:987–996.

19. Carpenter JL, Bachrach A Jr, Albert DM, Vainisi SJ, Goldstein MA. Xanthomatous keratitis, disseminated xanthomatosis, and atherosclerosis in Cuban tree frogs. Vet Pathol 1986;23: 337–339.

20. Keller CB, Shilton CM. The amphibian eye. Vet Clin N Am Exotic Anim Pract 2002;5: 261–274.

21. Xie ZY, Zhou YC, Wang SF, Mei B, Xu XD, Wen WY, Feng YQ. First isolation and identification of *Elizabethkingia meningoseptica* from cultured tiger frog, *Rana tigerina rugulosa*. Vet Microbiol 2009;138:140–144.

22. Brooks DE, Jacobson ER, Wolf ED, Clubb S, Gaskin JM. Panophthalmitis and otitis interna in fire-bellied toads. J Am Vet Med Assoc 1983;183:1198–1201.

23. Olson ME, Gard S, Brown M, Hampton R, Morck DW. *Flavobacterium indologenes* infection in leopard frogs. J Am Vet Med Assoc 1992;201:1766–1770.

24. Imai DM, Nadler SA, Brenner D, Donovan TA, Pessier AP. Rhabditid nematode-associated ophthalmitis and meningoencephalomyelitis in captive Asian horned frogs (*Megophrys montana*). J Vet Diagn Invest 2009;21:568–573.

25. Shen DF, Chang MA, Matteson DM, Buggage R, Kozhich AT, Chan CC. Biphasic ocular inflammatory response to endotoxin-induced uveitis in the mouse. Arch Ophthalmol 2000;118: 521–527.
26. Scheid P, Siffert W. Effects of inhibiting carbonic anhydrase on isometric contraction of frog skeletal muscle. J Physiol 1985;361:91–101.

# Chapter 12

# The fish eye

## Introduction

We said at the beginning of this volume that, in so many words, an eye... is an eye... is an eye. Even though they belong to animals inhabiting very different ecological niches, the basic anatomy, physiology and function of the eye is very similar across vertebrate species. If we had to pick one group, however, where this adaptation to their environment had given a substantially different set of features, this would have to be the fish. The underwater environment rules out the cornea having any refractive power and thus the fish lens is spherical. The light underwater is considerably different from that above water both in its spectral characteristics and its intensity. And the behavioural visual requirements are substantially different from those of animals on land. We will see how this influences piscine ocular anatomy and physiology in one moment but we also need to discuss briefly the way in which fish are kept in captivity, as this has a significant influence on their ocular health and disease.

The intimate contact between the ocular surface and the aqueous environment inhabited by fish renders deficiencies in that environment very important. Too high a build-up of bacteria or parasites in the water through inadequate filtering and water changes, incorrect pH or abnormally high levels of chemicals such as ammonia and nitrates, inadequate (or even excessive) oxygen concentrations, abnormal temperature and a host of other more minor factors can all adversely affect aquarium or pond fish health and this includes the eye as much as any other part of the body. A history taken before examining a fish with eye problems should thus make careful note of the state of the facility and its management as well as conditions of other in-contact fish. Perhaps more than in any other species group, interactions of the eye with the rest of the body and with the outside environment are particularly crucial.

Protection of the ocular surface does not need to be as profound as in animals where the corneal surface has to cope with air currents and the hazards they bring; this yields differences in lacrimation, in corneal epithelial structure and function, and in the need, or rather lack of need, for eyelids. On the other hand fish have to be prepared for the osmotic challenge of salt or fresh water, or even in some cases such as the daring salmon or the common eel, rapid transition between the two media. The lens must provide the

*Ophthalmology of Exotic Pets*, First Edition. David L. Williams.
© 2012 David Williams. Published 2012 by Blackwell Publishing Ltd.

entire refractive capability of the eye as the cornea underwater provides none. In the posterior segment the piscine photoreceptors differ considerably to those of their land-dwelling cousins: they are often in more than one row, are continually generated from a stem cell population, and need to respond to light at very different wavelengths from those detected by terrestrial animals.

A full outline of piscine ophthalmology would include information on farmed fish such as trout and salmon, wild-caught fish such as tuna and fish with importance from a conservation perspective from the green sturgeon to the great white shark. Wider assessments of the fish eye in health and disease are available [1,2], but here we focus on species most likely to be kept in aquaria, both freshwater and marine, and the ocular problems which derive from their being kept in captivity.

## Anatomy and physiology of the fish eye

One of the problems of dealing with ocular disease in such a wide and diverse group as fish is that from an anatomical and physiological perspective as well from one focusing on disease and ocular pathology, it is very difficult to make generalisations that, by the very fact of spreading the net too wide, if one with forgive the pun, the important details of particular species are lost. One advantage of constraining ourselves to aquarium fish is that generally, with certain exceptions such as the megaophthalmic black moor goldfish, of which more below, the fish being dealt with have a simple, relatively primitive piscine eye without the remarkable adaptations seen in the eyes of deep sea fish or, at the other end of the spectrum, those such as *Anableps*, the four-eyed fish, which live half above and half below the water surface.

We can then say that the fish dealt with here most often have an anterio-posteriorly flattened globe without eyelids (Figure 12.1 and Figure 12.2), though these are also seen in cartilaginous fish such as sharks and rays. The eye has a thick cornea which, because of immersion in water of an approximately equivalent refractive index to the aqueous humour, plays no part in refraction of light as it would do in an animal living with its eye exposed to air rather than water. Marine fish will have a thinner cornea than do their freshwater counterparts. Yellow pigmentation in the corneas of some surface-living fish, together with iridescence, may serve as a sunscreen to limit glare. The corneal epithelium has a much more important role in preventing ingress of water into the piscine cornea than does its mammalian equivalent, rendering corneal ulceration more serious than it can be in more conventionally treated species.

The fish lens is spherical and placed much more anteriorly in the eye than in mammals, this serving to optimise refraction now that the lens is the only refracting element in the eye and also to maximise light collection in an environment where illumination is at a premium. The fish lens has the highest refractive index of any vertebrate, around 1.69. A gradient of refractive index through the lens minimises spherical aberration which would otherwise severely compromise image formation in a spherical lens. The lens has a nucleus, cortex and capsule, as in any mammal lens, but its sphericity renders it impossible to deform as occurs in accommodation with many other species groups. Lens movement in an anterior–posterior direction thus changes the plane of focus of the entire

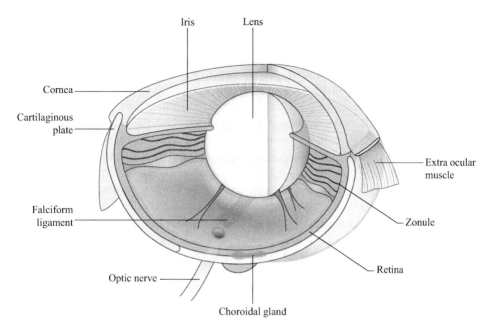

**Figure 12.1**  Line diagram of fish eye.

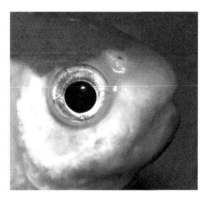

**Figure 12.2**  A normal goldfish eye. (Reproduced with permission from William Wildgoose.)

ocular imaging system. A dorsal suspensory ligament allows the lens to hang pendulum-like and be moved backwards and forwards by contraction and relaxation of the retractor lentis muscle. The retractor lentis muscle arises from the falciform ligament ventrally in the teleost (bony) fish eye. As its name suggests, the muscle pulls the lens, which normally sits within the pupil aperture, backwards to provide a shorter focal length. The cartilaginous sharks and rays, have an anterior protractor lentis muscle which does the exact opposite to vary the focusing power of the eye.

The uvea consists of iris, ciliary body and choroid, although the ciliary body appears rudimentary. The iris is heavily pigmented with an anterior stroma replete with guanophores in many species, giving the appearance of a metallic sheen to many fish irides. The pupil is often asymmetric and the anterior lens often protrudes through it, optimising light-gathering power. The iris has little in the way of musculature, either of the smooth or skeletal varieties and thus the pupil is for the most part stationary; the eye does not rely on pupillary constriction to limit light entry and pupillary light responses in fish are next to non-existent, an important factor to note in determining whether fish can see. The choroid, apart from acting as an immunological powerhouse of the posterior segment, plays a unique role in many fish species by which its choroidal rete, a tight-knit countercurrent system of blood vessels, can concentrate oxygen, particularly important in fish living in water with poor oxygen concentration, or at depth. This vascular network is connected to the pseudobranch or false gill in most teleost fish, an arrangement allowing high oxygen tensions to be delivered to the choroidal rete.

The piscine retina is highly unusual in that photoreceptors are continually added to its number. This relates to the continued growth in size of the eye through life, requiring the addition of rods in particular, but also means that if the retina becomes degenerate through cytotoxic effects, injury or surgical lesioning it can regenerate. Whether this is important in clinical retinal damage is unclear.

It was noted above that fish species do not generally rely on pupillary constriction to limit irradiation of the posterior segment of the eye. Instead the retina has two unique mechanisms through which it can vary the impact of light on its photoreceptors. The retinomotor response allows the photoreceptors to move in and out of recesses in the retinal pigment epithelium; cones move out of the protection of the retinal pigment epithelium in brighter light when their colour-vision responses are required while the rods move back into these protective retinal pigment epithelium sheaths. At night the opposite occurs so that photoreceptors with greater light sensitivity are more exposed in dim light conditions [1]. These changes take a matter of 1–2 hours to occur, an important factor to bear in mind if one is suddenly examining a fish eye with a bright light or bringing it into the light of an operating microscope to perform surgery. Phototoxic effects on the retina may give rise to a blind fish even if the rest of the surgery was successful.

## What do fish see?

Much has been written about the peculiarities of vision in the deep sea where the properties of down-welling light are very different from those on the surface. Yet as most of the pet fish we will deal with here are near-surface dwellers these considerations should not take much of our time here. The optics and visual capabilities of fish are covered in detail in the chapter on behavioural studies of fish vision in Douglas and Djamgoz' excellent volume *The Visual System of Fish* and readers are directed there for further information [2].

One might wonder why researchers would want to make the study of fish vision a priority. Yet in vision research for many years the goldfish retina has been an important model [3] and more recently the zebra danio (*Danio danio*) has provided an excellent primitive vertebrate model for transgenic investigation of the link between genotype and phenotype, with the eye being quite as well studied as other organ systems [4]. Thus zebra danio vision has been evaluated as a measure of retinal function, by use of the optokinetic response [5] and through behavioural responses which manifest early in larval development [6].

Visual sensitivity, the lowest light levels at which vision is still possible, vary considerably between different species living in different photic environments. It appears that the sensivity of goldfish vision equates to one photon absorbed per 15000 rods per second [7], the equivalent number in the human eye being 900 photic rhodopsin isomerisations per second. Clearly the goldfish eye, seeing in the lower light environment under water, is orders of magnitude more sensitive.

Visual acuity for goldfish has been determined as between 1.2 and 1.5 cycles per degree (cpd). Note that using Snellen acuity measures 20/20 is 30 cpd and 20/200 is 3 cpd so goldfish vision is around 20/400. But there are substantial cross-species differences in acuity, primarily for two reasons. First, the density of photoreceptors in the retina varies considerably across species; those relying on vision in environments of higher light intensity have more densely packed photoreceptors and thus higher acuity. Secondly fish with larger eyes have a great acuity, predominantly because larger lenses have less in the way of spherical and chromatic aberration but also because if the lens is further from the retina, the image size will be larger and resolution improved.

For a fish, in a continually moving visual environment, the detection of static images is of little importance compared with motion detection. Thus measuring critical flicker frequency (CFF), the temporal rather than spatial resolution of the eye, is important in fish. This can be achieved behaviourally or, more readily, by electroretinography. These again show a wide variation between species of between 4.4 and 95.8 Hz; again an active predatory fish has to have a higher CFF than a sedentary bottom feeder, and that is exactly what we find.

Colour vision again varies between species but the fact that water screens out shorter wavelength illumination means that the spectrum of light for which most fish respond is constricted at the blue end of the spectrum. Fish have four photoreceptor cones rather than the meagre three we humans possess; quite how this relates to behavioural responses is beyond the scope of this short discussion. Interestingly as well as differentiating light of different spectra, the fish eye responds to light differently polarised. Grasping what this means is almost impossible to us humans, blind to polarisation, but behavioural studies suggest that polarisation of downwelling solar illumination through water has a significant effect on fish motion in the short range and also quite possibly in migration, as indeed it may do for other taxa as varied as butterflies and birds.

Finally fish also have their lateral line system which gives then a totally novel sensory system allowing detection of objects in their close environment without the need for eyes. So we might ask, does vision matter in an aquarium environment where food is provided and migration impossible? Blind fish in aquaria generally have a lower food conversion ratio and smaller size. They may have more aggressive interactions with conspecifics as is certainly seen in some aquaculture environments. Vision in these animals certainly does matter, though conceivably in a different manner from that in terrestrial species. And so we come to discuss diseases of the fish eye, their diagnosis and treatment.

## Diseases of the aquarium fish eye

### Anophthalmos

#### Clinical signs

On occasion fish will be noted with congenital anophthalmos or lack of any ocular structures. In other fish trauma or infection can lead to loss of the globe in which case the dermal layers regenerate over the empty orbit yielding the appearance of anophthalmos. It is surprising how well such fish cope in an aquarium environment although their small size relative to sighted fellow tank dwellers shows their reduced food conversion ratio (Figure 12.3). Blinded individuals in commercial fish farms show a similarly limited growth rate.

#### Aetiopathogenesis

Some fish are congenitally anophthalmic or severely microphthalmic. In the blind cave fish *Astyanax mexicanus* ocular development starts but the embryonic ocular primordia degenerate. The lens disappears through apoptosis and subsequently the retina degenerates, retinal cells undergo apoptosis and retinal growth is arrested. In the sighted surface-dwelling form of the fish the eye develops normally [8]. Another example of anophthalmos in fish is the el (eyeless) mutation in medaka (*Oryzias latipes*), a recessive mutation which affects eye formation; in the most severe cases it results in the absence of eyes with small optic cup-like structures differentiating in situ in the walls of the prosencephalon without the evagination which usually forms the eye cups. Anophthalmic fish hatch normally but do not respond to visual stimuli and in the small fraction which grow to adulthood the brain exhibits a number of abnormalities [9].

The mechanism by which trauma can lead to apparent anophthalmos, unilaterally or bilaterally is unclear.

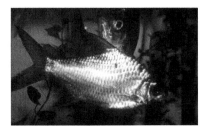

**Figure 12.3**   Bilaterally anophthalmic fish after trauma.

## **Macrophthalmos**

### *Clinical signs*

A number of goldfish strains (*Carassius auratus*) are characterised by enlarged eyes, the most common of these being the black moor (Figure 12.4), the subject of some considerable research on the mechanisms of abnormal globe enlargement [10]. These animals have visual eyes, though highly myopic ones and an ocular surface which, because of its protruding nature, is often the site of traumatic injury. Indeed the lifespan of these animals in a normal aquarium is generally considerably shorter than that of a conventional goldfish cohort. Other goldfish strains such as the bubble eye, have enlarged lymph-filled sacs in the infraorbital region (Figure 12.5) and while these might be mistaken for globe enlargement at first sight, a closer inspection will show that the 'bubble' is adnexal and not ocular in origin. While trauma can lead to puncture of these sacs they usually reinflate with time.

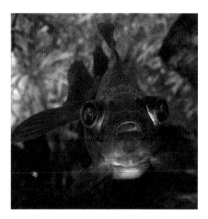

**Figure 12.4**   Black moor goldfish with protuberant eyes.

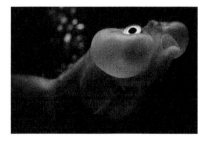

**Figure 12.5**   Bubble eye goldfish with infraorbital lymph-filled sacs.

### Aetiopathogenesis

The exact gene or genes leading to the development of these enlarged globes is unclear. The myopia is caused through vitreal chamber enlargement and not through abnormal lens development [11].

## Exophthalmos ('pop eye')

### Clinical signs

Exophthalmos is considered by many to be the most prevalent ocular disorder in aquarium fish [12]. Orbital anatomy in teleost fish means that a relatively small space-occupying lesion in the retrobulbar area, or indeed expansion of the posterior segment of the globe, produces a pronounced forward movement of the globe.

The signs seen concurrent with exophthalmos in land-dwelling mammalian species, such as lagophthalmos, failure of complete eyelid closure with subsequent exposure keratitis are not seen in fish with exophthalmos, but predisposition to trauma is increased and vision may be compromised.

### Aetiopathogenesis

A large number of factors may be involved in the development of exophthalmos in fish from trauma, environmental influences such as oxygen supersaturation giving gas bubble disease, infectious organisms from viruses to parasites, dietary deficiencies or neoplasia (Figure 12.6).

Gas bubble disease is most commonly caused by increased levels of dissolved gases (nitrogen or oxygen normally increased in partial pressure through gas being intrained into water in a faulty pumping system). This occurs predominantly in aquaculture systems but can be seen in aquaria for pet fish also. The dissolved gases form gas bubbles in the vasculature of the fish including the gills and skin but most obviously appreciated in the

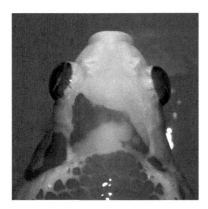

**Figure 12.6**   A goldfish with exophthalmos or 'pop eye' from systemic tuberculosis. (Reproduced with permission from William Wildgoose.)

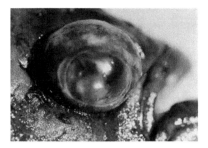

**Figure 12.7** Enlarged and exophthalmic eye from choroidal gas bubble formation.

countercurrent mechanisms of the choroidal gland, thus resulting in exophthalmos (Figure 12.7).

Swim bladder inflammation is seen with a number of infectious organisms giving a systemic vasculitis, again most commonly appreciated with engorgement of the vessels of the choroidal gland with subsequent exophthalmos.

### Clinical management

Treatment of these cases clearly relies on an understanding of what factors underlie the retrobulbar lesion.

If gas bubbles are seen under the skin, in the gills or within the eye, and the fish is kept in a supersaturated environment, remedying the dissolved oxygen levels using a commercial water degasser is critical but not generally sufficient to resolve the problem. Use of carbonic anhydrase inhibitors may resolve choroidal gas bubbles with a peribulbar injection of 6 mg/kg acetazolamide being reported as successful. However, systemic absorption of the drug can give problems with gas transport in another rete, that of the swimbladder gas gland where dysfunction gives buoyancy problems. Topical carbonic anhydrase inhibitors such as dorzolamide in Trusopt would give fewer systemic effects but success with their use has not been reported in the literature.

If choroidal gland enlargement is associated with an infection then ameliorative treatment with systemic antibiosis may be effective but again once the globe has been displaced anteriorly there is little that can be done to resolve the problem and the attention must switch to in-contact animals to ensure that the same pathology does not occur in these fish.

### Corneal ulceration: ulcerative keratitis

### Clinical signs

Corneal ulceration is a common condition in aquarium fish and most commonly occurs after trauma (Figure 12.8). Retention of fluorescein stain is, as with any animal with a corneal ulcer, the definitive proof of the lesion and this test can be performed with the fish out of water for a few moments. Some suggest that the animal is held in a damp

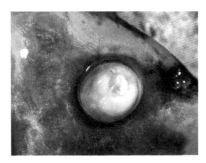

**Figure 12.8**   Corneal ulceration with oedema in a goldfish. (Reproduced with permission from William Wildgoose.)

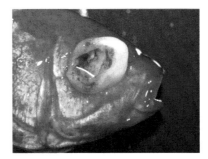

**Figure 12.9**   Keratitis and panophthalmitis with globe collapse. (Reproduced with permission from William Wildgoose.)

towel but the risk of skin or eye damage requires anaesthesia of such a fish with MS222 or benzocaine. The difference between corneal ulceration in the fish from that in land-based vertebrates is the propensity to develop profound corneal oedema. The earliest signs of an epithelial abrasion are an oval edge of damaged epithelium but very rapidly the ulcer bed becomes grey and oedematous. Development and worsening of the ulcer can occur rapidly and thus it may be at the point of corneal perforation and globe rupture that the fish is presented.

### Aetiopathogenesis

The lack of eyelids in all teleost fish render the ocular surface highly prone to traumatic insult, be this from aquarium 'furniture' or attacks by other fish. Commercial fish farms recognise this 'eye snapping' by aggressive individuals at feeding time. This is less of a problem in most aquarium fish, except for those bred specifically for an aggressive temperament, such as Japanese fighting fish *Betta splendens*. Thus the vast majority of piscine corneal ulcers start as a superficial abrasion; the rapid onset of corneal oedema and the presence of infectious organisms in the water of a less than perfectly maintained aquarium, lead to deepening of the corneal ulcer with potential globe perforation and subsequent endophthalmitis (Figure 12.9).

Bacterial skin disease, especially with organisms such as *Cytophaga* or *Flavobacter* can extend to cause ocular surface disease and the rest of the animal should always be examined where corneal ulceration is present.

## Clinical management

Because of the potential for rapid worsening of corneal ulcers in aquarium fish, treatment should be instituted as rapidly as possible. The likelihood that normal commensal organisms on the surface of the fish may become pathogens in the exposed oedematous corneal stroma means that prophylactic antibiosis is essential. While it might be thought that obtaining diagnostic samples for bacteriology would be useful, a skin swab probably yields no more information than a water sample. Bacteriology probably should be retained for circumstances where antibiosis has not been successful. A cytology specimen may be useful; this is harvested with a cytobrush applied to the corneal surface and used to produce an air-dried smear on a slide for a modified Giemsa stain.

A 10-day bath in furazone green at 0.017 g/l has been suggested as appropriate in superficial ulcers [13]; this topical treatment contains monofuracin, furazolidone and methylene blue giving antibacterial and antifungal action, but is only available currently in the USA. Sodium chloride, added to the water at 1–2 g/l can be beneficial for freshwater fish and has a mild antiseptic action while also reducing the osmotic gradient across the skin. Deeper ulcers likely to perforate may be treated with cyanoacrylate glue allowed to dry for 1–2 minutes while the fish is maintained in a hydrated state out of the tank, anaesthetised and ventilated with oxygenated water through the gills. Such a glue will only adhere to a dry corneal surface and thus dessication of the ulcer bed is vital before applying the adhesive – use of cotton-tipped applicators or better still an air-jet similar to those used to clear dust from photographic negatives is useful in this regard. Postoperative treatment should include an antibiotic bath as detailed above while the underlying cornea heals and eventually the adhesive layer lifts off the corneal surface.

As noted above all too many ulcers progress rapidly to descemetocoeles where only Descemet's membrane remains between an intact cornea and a perforated globe. In these cases use of cyanoacrylate adhesive is probably not to be recommended as the exothermic reaction can cause further damage and globe rupture.

In all cases it is vital to maintain water quality especially with regard to sterility – use of ozone in a separate bubble chamber or ultraviolet irradiation to remove pathogens from the water during filtration should be considered where bacterial keratitis appears as a frequent problem in in-contact fish.

## Non-ulcerative keratitis

### Clinical signs

Interstitial keratitis may manifest as corneal opacification with oedema, cellular infiltrates appearing as a grey haze together with fibroplasia as a more pronounced opacification of the cornea. In such cases there will be no immediate uptake of fluorescein

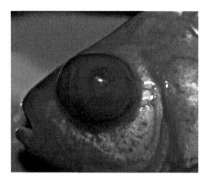

**Figure 12.10**   Keratitis following exposure and trauma in a goldfish. (Reproduced with permission from William Wildgoose.)

as seen in ulcerative keratitis but after a few minutes a diffuse granular uptake may be noted. While this does not denote frank loss of epithelium, it suggests that the corneal epithelium, while still in place, has lost the integrity of its intercellular tight junctions (Figure 12.10).

### Aetiopathogenesis

A number of causes from infectious agents to environmental factors such as excess ultraviolet light or even nutritional deficiencies in vitamin A, thiamine or riboflavin can lead to corneal opacification. Parasites normally found on the skin may also involve the corneal surface with the most common ones being *Glugea* or *Icththyophthirius* while trematodes, anchorworms and lice have been reported as causing ocular surface pathology, although generally in commercial fisheries not aquarium stock.

### Clinical management

Often corneal opacification through such influences can be very difficult to resolve, since the damage is already done once the aetiological factors have been identified. Preventing further exposure to these will halt the progress of the condition and prevent other in-contact fish being affected, but often cannot reverse the signs in the first fish affected.

### Cataract

### Clinical signs

Lens opacities in fish, whether farmed commercially or in aquarium settings, are all too common (Figure 12.11). Cataracts can progress rapidly to a fully mature white lens and it may be only at this stage that the pathology is noted, while closer examination with

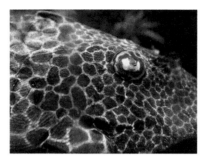

**Figure 12.11**  Cataract in a *Hypostomus* suckerfish.

equipment such as a slit lamp biomicroscope can show earlier changes in the lens which do not fully obscure vision.

## Aetiopathogenesis

A number of different factors can cause cataract formation in fish. Excess ultraviolet light may be an influence in a surface-dwelling species while nutritional deficiency can be a cause in any species. This is surprisingly common and very important in commercial fish farms but perhaps less so in aquarium fish. Poor water quality may give rise to cataracts through osmotic changes in the lens. Cataract was noted in a number of wolf fish after an increase in water temperature [14]; cataracts have also been noted in fish subjected to freezing temperatures, this more likely to take place in animals kept in an outside aquarium or a garden pond than ones living in an indoor tank.

A common cause of cataracts is the involvement of trematode flukes, particularly the species *Diplostomum* which embed themselves in the lens. This may seem an unusual place for such a parasite to reside but studies have shown that fish thus blinded swim near the surface and thus are more likely to be predated by birds which are the definitive host for the parasite.

## Clinical management

Cataracts can be removed from the fish eye in the same way that surgery is performed in more conventional species by phacoemulsification. It has been suggested that the fish lens is considerably more dense than that of a mammal rendering removal by phacoemulsification more difficult [11]. Only one report appears to exist in the literature concerning phacoemulsification in a fish and in that no mention was made of surgery being more difficult than in a dog or cat [15]. Indeed that report documented removal of a lens in which the cataract was caused by migrating *Diplostomum* larvae.

Other measures taken against this cataractogenic trematode include a 1–3-hour bath in praziquantel (Droncit, Bayer) at 2 mg/l repeated after 7 and 14 days. The problem here is that the anthelmintic kills the larvae with the potential for a substantial immune response against dead and dying larvae with ensuing panophthalmitis.

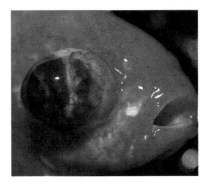

**Figure 12.12**   Panophthalmitis in a goldfish. (Reproduced with permission from William Wildgoose.)

### *Uveitis*

#### *Clinical signs*

Anterior uveitis presents in fish with signs similar to those in mammals – episcleral hyperaemia, corneal oedema, aqueous flare manifest as a haziness of iris detail, synechiae or adhesions of the pupil margin to the anterior lens capsule and, most obviously, hyphaema or hypopyon, blood or purulent exudate respectively, in the anterior chamber of the eye. The small size most fish eyes and the association of many cases of uveitis with systemic infectious disease (see further below) means that the most common presenting signs of uveitis involve inflammation of all structures within the eye, so-called panophthalmitis (Figure 12.12). In some cases the inflammatory damage can be so severe that the globe becomes phthytic, reducing in size until only the skin-covered orbit remains, a process we might call inflammatory enucleation.

#### *Aetiopathogenesis*

A number of different causes may result in intraocular inflammation from trauma, through helminth migration and *Myxobolus* infection or bacterial infection. This is the case not only with localised infection but also, and probably more commonly, as a result of septicaemia either with Gram-negative bacteria, such as *Aeromonas* and *Pseudomonas*, or less frequently Gram-positive organisms, such as *Staphylococcus* or *Streptococcus*. Even uveal neoplasms can give rise to intraocular inflammation (Figure 12.13).

#### *Clinical management*

As with exophthalmos, uveitis often signals a systemic disease which requires a wider assessment of the animal as a whole. Other signs of infection may be seen, such as dermal petechiae, raised scales, dropsy (accumulation of fluid in the body cavity), lethargy or anorexia. All these are signs that the ocular inflammation is merely part of a more generalised condition. Uveitis is so often associated with septicaemia that a blood culture

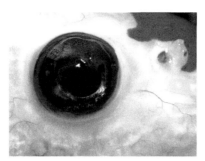

**Figure 12.13**   Uveitis associated with uveal neoplasm in a goldfish. (Reproduced with permission from William Wildgoose.)

can be useful, although where keratitis is also involved a bacteriological and cytological sample of the ocular surface will be valuable to detect bacterial and viral conditions. Treatment of the eye is difficult but improving the water quality and potentially treating any systemic bacterial disease with baths of sodium chloride or malachite green can be appropriate.

## Retinal disease

### Clinical signs

It is unusual to note changes such as chorioretinitis or retinal detachment without looking for them specifically with an ophthalmoscope. Even then, as we noted above, ophthalmoscopy to view the retina is difficult because of the degree of corneal curvature and the spherical nature of the lens. Rendering the corneal surface flat with a microscope cover-slip can be helpful.

### Aetiopathogenesis

Retinal inflammation or detachment is often part of panophthalmitis, although a diabetic retinopathy has been reported in carp. Adenocarcinoma of the retinal pigment epithelium and retinoblastoma have been reported but these neoplasms are likely only to be found at a post-mortem examination unless ultrasonography is employed to define them.

### Clinical management

Given that retinal disease in fish is generally associated with intraocular inflammation, treatment of the ensuing panophthalmitis generally requires systemic antibiotic and anti-inflammatory medication given for such disease. Globe removal can be performed in such cases [16,17]. Another reason for enucleation can be to perform a transorbital hypophysectomy [18].

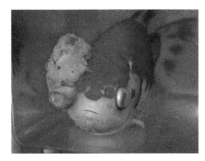

**Figure 12.14**   Fibroma in a goldfish. (Reproduced with permission from William Wildgoose.)

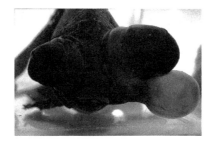

**Figure 12.15**   Retinal pigment epithelial carcinoma in a black moor goldfish. (Reproduced with permission from William Wildgoose.)

### *Neoplasia*

#### *Clinical signs*

Space-occupying tumours can arise in any part of the eye, with varying clinical signs, so a retrobulbar mass gives exophthalmos and eventually extrusion of the neoplasm from the orbit (Figure 12.14). Uveal neoplasms are often manifest through a glaucomatous globe enlargement but before that may be visualised as a mass in the iris. Posterior segment tumours such as retinoblastoma, retinal pigment epithelial carcinoma (Figure 12.15) and medulloepitheliosarcoma are very interesting from a comparative pathology perspective but are rarely seen in aquarium fish medicine; they all give rise to globe enlargement and blindness.

#### *Aetiopathogenesis*

As with neoplasms in any species, ocular tumours in fish may be caused by genetic mutations or by environmental influences. In the majority of cases of ocular neoplasia in aquarium fish an aetiopathology cannot be determined.

## Clinical management

While enucleation might be considered worthwhile in a valuable koi carp or similar fish, in most cases the welfare of the fish is best served by euthanasia, normally with an overdose of intracoelomic barbiturate.

# References

1. Fernald RD. Vision. In: Evans DH, ed. *The Physiology of Fishes*. Boca Raton, LA: CRC Press, 1993; pp. 161–189.
2. Douglas R, Djamgoz M. *The Visual System of Fish*. London: Chapman and Hall, 1990.
3. Kaneko A. Physiological studies of single retinal cells and their morphological identification. Vision Res 1971;Suppl 3:17–26.
4. Bilotta J, Saszik S. The zebrafish as a model visual system. Int J Dev Neurosci 2001;19: 621–629.
5. Huang YY, Neuhauss SC. The optokinetic response in zebrafish and its applications. Front Biosci 2008;13:1899–1916.
6. Neuhauss SC. Behavioral genetic approaches to visual system development and function in zebrafish. J Neurobiol 2003;54:148–160.
7. Powers MK, Easter SS. Absolute visual sensitivity of the goldfish. Vision Res 1978;18: 1149–1154.
8. Tian NM, Price DJ. Why cavefish are blind. Bioessays 2005;27:235–238.
9. Ishikawa Y, Yoshimoto M, Yamamoto N, Ito H, Yasuda T, Tokunaga F, Iigo M, Wakamatsu Y, Ozato K. Brain structures of a medaka mutant, el (eyeless), in which eye vesicles do not evaginate. Brain Behav Evol 2001;58:173–184.
10. Easter SS Jr, Hitchcock PF. The myopic eye of the Black Moor goldfish. Vision Res 1986;26: 1831–1833.
11. Seltner RL, Weerheim JA, Sivak JG. Role of the lens and vitreous humor in the refractive properties of the eyes of three strains of goldfish. Vision Res 1989;29:681–685.
12. Jurj I. Ophthalmic disease of fish. Vet Clin N Am 2002;5:243–260.
13. Williams CR, Whitaker BR. The evaluation and treatment of common ocular disorders in Teleosts. Sem Av Ex Pet Med 1997;6:160–169.
14. Bjerkås E, Bjerkås I, Moksness E. An outbreak of cataract with lens rupture and nuclear extrusion in wolf-fish (*Anarhicas* spp.). Vet Ophthalmol 1998;1:9–15.
15. Bakal RS, Hickson BH, Gilger BC, Levy MG, Flowers JR, Khoo L. Surgical removal of cataracts due to *Diplostomum* species in Gulf sturgeon (*Acipenser oxyrinchus desotoi*). J Zoo Wildl Med 2005;36:504–508.
16. Wildgoose W. Exenteration in fish. Exotic DVM 2007;9:25–29.
17. Nadelstein B, Bakal R, Lewbart GA. Orbital exenteration and placement of a prosthesis in fish. J Am Vet Med Assoc 1997;211: 603–606.
18. Nishioka RS, Richman NH, Young G, Prunet P, Bern HA. Hypophysectomy of coho salmon (*Oncorhynchus kisutch*) and survival in fresh water and seawater. Aquaculture 1987;65: 343–352.

# Conclusions

We said at the beginning of this volume that the eye varied surprisingly little between species, yet had sufficient diversity to render specific attention to the differences important. I hope that the layout of the text has allowed sufficient discussion of these differences at an academic level while focusing on the clinical diagnosis and management of ocular disease across the species range. Some diseases, such as corneal ulceration, span the species divide, yet others, such as diseases of the snake spectacle, are very specific to that group of animals. These latter conditions are more difficult for veterinarians to identify as they present relatively infrequently. Indeed one of the problems with dealing with exotic species as a generalist, is that their particular peculiarities are not commonly encountered in routine veterinary practice. I wonder if, following on from that thought, I might be permitted a moment to ponder what this book has shown me philosophically about keeping some of these exotic pets in captivity. The fact that we may encounter species such as reptiles or primates relatively infrequently means that we do not have an innate sense of what they are feeling, as we might have with a dog or cat.

Take the rabbit we saw in Chapter 4 with a lymphoma obstructing its cranial venous drainage which develops exophthalmos when handled. We happily noted with fascination that raised arterial blood pressure and impaired venous drainage leads to an engorgement of the retrobulbar venous plexus with subsequent globe protrusion. But what does that say about what the rabbit feels about being handled? As a prey species is has evolved to exhibit what we might call 'learned helplessness' but maybe its eyes and the momentary hypertension they reveal show us in this one instance what it really is feeling deep inside. Take the slender lorises in Chapter 8 where treatment was more problematic than the dry eye affecting them – a dog with KCS accepts regular medication from its owner because of the bond that exists between them, but by the very nature of being exotic many of these animals are not amenable to regular treatment. What does that tell us about the ethics of keeping them in the first place?

Having said that, there would be no reason for writing this book if treatment of ocular disease in these species was impossible or if keeping them in captivity was entirely unethical. Our aim should be to optimise their welfare and that must mean providing the best ophthalmic diagnostic and therapy we can. I do hope that this volume will provide readily available information which will aid in diagnosis and treatment of eye disease

*Ophthalmology of Exotic Pets*, First Edition. David L. Williams.
© 2012 David Williams. Published 2012 by Blackwell Publishing Ltd.

from amphibians to zebrafish and as well will provoke more interest in the fascinating subject of comparative visual physiology and behaviour.

I have to thank so many people, both ophthalmologists and exotic animal clinicians, for help over the years in understanding these animals and their eyes more and more. Writing this book has shown me how much I still have to learn and I hope that those with greater experience and knowledge than I will forgive errors and omissions along the way. I am always happy to be contacted by e-mail through my website www. davidlwilliams.org.uk so please do send comments and corrections to me there!

# Index

*Ophthalmology of Exotic Pets*, First Edition. David L. Williams.
© 2012 David Williams. Published 2012 by Blackwell Publishing Ltd.

Printed and bound by CPI Group (UK) Ltd, Croydon, CR0 4YY

27/10/2024

14580388-0001